HEALTH INEQUALITY:
MORALITY AND MEASUREMENT

YUKIKO ASADA

Health Inequality

Morality and Measurement

UNIVERSITY OF TORONTO PRESS
Toronto Buffalo London

© University of Toronto Press Incorporated 2007
Toronto Buffalo London
Printed in Canada

ISBN 978-0-8020-9244-1

∞

Printed on acid-free paper

Library and Archives Canada Cataloguing in Publication

Asada, Yukiko
Health inequality : morality and measurement / Yukiko Asada.

Includes bibliographical references and index.
ISBN 978-0-8020-9244-1

1. Equality – Health aspects.   2. Public health – Moral and ethical aspects.
3. Public health – Social aspects.   4. Health services accessibility.
5. Equality – Health aspects – United States.   I. Title.

RA418.A83 2007   362.1′042   C2007-905114-6

This book has been published with the help of a grant from the Nova Scotia
Health Research Foundation, through the Knowledge Transfer (Exchange)
Award in the Research Capacity Awards Program.

University of Toronto Press acknowledges the financial assistance to its
publishing program of the Canada Council for the Arts and the Ontario Arts
Council.

University of Toronto Press acknowledges the financial support for its
publishing activities of the Government of Canada through the
Book Publishing Industry Development Program (BPIDP).

To my parents, Ken and Hiroko Asada

Contents

Figures and Tables

Figures

Tables

Acknowledgments

This project began on a rainy day in January 2000 in Geneva, Switzerland. I was starting a four-month internship in the Program on Evidence for Health Policy at the World Health Organization following the appointment of my PhD co-supervisor, Dan Wikler, as the first staff ethicist for the WHO. Little did I know on that day that *The World Health Report 2000* would define my internship and health inequality would become a topic that would fascinate me for the coming years. Albeit with no involvement, for the next four months I witnessed the exciting development of the WHO health inequality index for *The World Health Report 2000*. Emmanuela Gakidou, Chris Murray, Julio Frenk, and David Evans immensely stimulated my thinking. I am often critical of the approach taken for the WHO health inequality index in this book, but its strong influence on my thinking is undeniable. It was also during these four months that Larry Temkin's book *Inequality* came to my attention. As much as I love my work, it is rare to find an academic page-turner for which I would eagerly sacrifice sleep. *Inequality* was such a book to me. I would like to thank Larry for his inspiration, and later, his comments on my specific questions to develop chapter 4 of this book.

Following the internship at the WHO, this project found three academic homes during its development. First, the Department of Population Health Sciences at the University of Wisconsin–Madison provided me with foundational education and a vision for truly multidisciplinary population health work. My deepest gratitude goes to the dissertation committee members, who enthusiastically supported the dissertation from which this book is derived. I thank Dan Wikler for his vision for population-level bioethics and his inspiration and encouragement, first to enter the PhD program in population health with an interest in ethics, and later to commit myself to the topic of health inequality. I am deeply indebted to Dave Kindig and John Mullahy for their unfailing support in every possible way for this project. As for many other students, after taking Dave's course on social determinants of health, the world looked different to me. I take pride in his comment on this work: 'This is truly a population health project.' I was privileged to have Dan Hausman guide me, with patience and intellectual rigour, to philosophical thinking of equality and justice. Without his constant encouragement and belief in this project, this book would not have existed. I am also thankful to Pat Remington and Alberto Palloni for their insightful suggestions, which frequently opened my eyes to new ways of thinking. Other individuals in Wisconsin who helped me shape my ideas include Denny Fryback, Maureen Smith, Mari Palta, Bobbi Wolfe, Terry Young, Tasha Stout, Hong Wang, Chris Seplaki, Thomas Hedemann, Indiana Strombom, Nilay Shah, Ben Craig, Ralph Insinga, Henry (Joe) Henk, Kirstie Danielson, Hana Said, and Elizabeth Cox.

This project's second and third homes were the Department of Bioethics and the Department of Community Health and Epidemiology, both at Dalhousie University. I would like to thank members of these departments for their warm acceptance of my unusual combination of interests in ethics and quantitative methods. In particular, Nuala Kenny, Susan Sherwin, and Sharon Batt consistently pressed me to clarify my arguments, and George Kephart constantly encouraged me with his belief in the value of multidisciplinary work.

In addition to people at these three places, the project benefited from the following individuals. Yasushi Ohkusa helped and guided the health inequality analysis in Japan from which empirical analyses in this book derive. Ole Frithjof Norheim provided very helpful comments for chapter 4. I am also grateful to the staff at the University of Toronto Press. In particular, Virgil Duff and Anne Laughlin, my editors, provided effective assistance throughout the process of book making; Charles Stuart, my copy-editor, helped improve the presentation of my thoughts; and anonymous ex-ternal reviewers gave me constructive suggestions. In addition, Ingrid Sketris, Joy Calkin, and members of the Network for End of Life Studies offered helpful advice on how to secure financial sources to publish this book. Questions and comments provided by my friends and colleagues have helped me to present my ideas much more fully than I might otherwise have done. All remaining errors are mine.

Over the years generous financial support from various sources made this project possible. I would like to thank the Fulbright Scholarship, the United States Agency for Healthcare Research and Quality's dissertation award (grant number 1 R03 HS13116), a post-doctoral fellowship in the ethics of health research and policy supported by the Canadian Institutes of Health Research, and the Nova Scotia Health Research Foundation for the financial assistance to publish this book. Part of chapter 1 appeared as 'Is health inequality across individuals of moral concern?' in *Health Care Analysis* 14, no. 1: 25–36 in 2006, and part of chapter 3 appeared as 'Medical technologies, nonhuman aids, human assistance, and environmental factor in the assessment of health states' in *Quality of Life Research* 14, no. 3: 867–74 in 2005. I thank Springer Science and Business Media for kind permission to use.

Finally, I would like to give a few personal notes. My husband, Brook Taylor, patiently and with constant encouragement, served as a sounding board for the ideas expressed in this project when they were still haphazardly arranged in my brain and read all chapters many times. He has my deep appreciation for his patience, understanding, and trust in my ability to carry out the work. I am deeply grateful for my parents' trust in me and courage to let me pursue my will. My philosophical study of equality started with them in their equitable treatment to my brothers and me based on their equal respect for each of us. I dedicate this book to my parents, who eagerly await a Japanese translation.

HEALTH INEQUALITY:
MORALITY AND MEASUREMENT

1 Introduction

1.1 Setting the Stage

Let us start this book by thinking about inequality in general. Although the notion of inequality can sometimes have moral connotations, for this book, at the outset, let us adopt the simplest definition of the word: 'the state or condition of being unequal' – that is, 'not the same in any measurable aspect, such as extent or quantity.'[1] Inequality is everywhere – the length of hair is surely different among your co-workers (unless you are a monk), the income of each household of your apartment building is likely to vary, your town probably includes people with different cultural backgrounds, the park in your neighbourhood is filled with different kinds of plants and animals, and Mars apparently has grains of sand of different sizes.

Among these ubiquitous inequalities, we are interested in some and do not care about others. Inequality in the size of grains of sand on Mars, for example, might be scientifically interesting. Inequality in the length of hair among employees in one's company, on the other hand, is unlikely to provoke any curiosity. Some inequalities are not only interesting but also invite judgment as to goodness and badness. We worry about some inequalities, for example, income inequality within and between nations. We do not, however, worry that different kinds of plants and animals live in a park. On the contrary, we appreciate such difference and have coined a special term for it, 'biodiversity.' We are ambivalent about the goodness and badness of some inequalities. For example, some countries like Canada generally appreciate multiculturalism, while other counties like Japan prefer to be homogeneous.

Inequality is everywhere, but only certain inequalities worry us.

Indeed, no one would wish equality in everything among everybody everywhere. As Kurt Vonnegut Jr magnificently depicts in his classic short story 'Harrison Bergeron,' perfect equality in 'every which way' would be a horror (Vonnegut 1950).[2]

Among the ubiquitous inequalities, what kind of inequality is *health* inequality? Is it the kind of inequality that interests us? If so, in what way? Do we make any judgment on the goodness and badness of health inequality?

Health inequality has long attracted keen attention in research and policy arenas. The history of the documentation of health inequality by social class in the United Kingdom, for example, goes back 150 years (Acheson 1998). It started with the first census in 1853 (Acheson 1998; Deaton 2002). Health inequality has now clearly established itself as a thriving research topic in various academic fields.[3]

Academics and policy-makers have recognized that health inequality is not merely an academic topic but has important policy implications. Among the documentation of health inequality by social class in the United Kingdom, researchers consider the 1980 Report of the Working Group on Inequalities in Health, commonly known as *The Black Report* (Black et al. 1992), a landmark document.[4] *The Black Report* is notable because it is a product of the government's formal enquiry into health inequality. The chairperson, Sir Douglas Black, along with members of the Working Group of Inequalities in Health, confirmed the speculation circulating around the time of this enquiry that health inequality by social class had not only persisted but widened during the first thirty years of the establishment of the National Health System. *The Black Report* summarized scattered evidence of health inequality by social class and made policy recommendations on how to address this problem.

Since *The Black Report*, several important policy documents on health inequality have been published in the UK. It was only in the late 1990s, however, that the political will existed to tackle health inequality. In 1997 the new Labour government appointed the Scientific Advisory Group on the Independent Inquiry into Inequalities in Health to summarize evidence on health inequality in the UK and to identify policy priorities. The resulting report, known as *The Acheson Report* (Acheson 1998), provided the basis for a three-year policy plan for reducing health inequality in the UK (UK Department of Health 2003). The British government is seriously concerned about evidence such as the widening mortality gap between professionals and unskilled workers. The mortality rate for unskilled workers was 1.2 times greater than for professionals in 1930–2; by 1991–3 the gap had increased to 2.9 times (Acheson 1998). The government aims at a concrete target of 'by 2010 reducing inequalities in health outcomes by 10 per cent as measured by infant mortality and life expectancy at birth' through the commitment to the inter-sectorial approach (UK Department of Health 2003, 7).

In Canada, the issue of health inequality has grown in importance as the concept of population health has gained credence among researchers and policy-makers. The population health perspective is concerned with the question of why some populations are healthier than others and emphasizes multiple determinants of health beyond the single factor of health care. The population health perspective has evolved since 1974, when the then minister of health Marc Lalonde emphasized the importance of multiple determinants of health in *A New Perspective on the Health of Canadians* (1974). Since then it has penetrated health research and policy in Canada. The federal, provincial, and territorial ministers of health, for example, officially adopted the population health concept in 1994, and Health Canada promotes the concept as one of its four priority areas (Health Canada 1996). Although policy action towards reducing health inequality in Canada may not be as dynamic as it is in the UK, the widespread acceptance of the population health concept suggests that Canadians are committed to reducing health inequality.

Even the United States, whose market-oriented health care system may not suggest an image of a benevolent society concerned about health inequality, is no stranger to concerns about health inequality. Inequalities in health care and health outcome by race or ethnicity have long been a major policy concern in that country.[5] In addition, a substantial number of policy initiatives in the United States have been directed towards addressing health inequality by socio-economic status (SES), paralleling to some extent research into and policy on health inequality by social class in Britain. A growing interest in health inequality in U.S. health policy is evident in *Healthy People 2010*, the national health plan for the first decade of the twenty-first century (U.S. Department of Health and Human Services 2000). Similar to the acceptance of the population health concept in Canada, it clearly sets two goals: increasing quality and years of healthy life, and eliminating health disparities.

The policy influence does not stop at the national level but extends internationally. The World Health Organization (WHO) Regional Office for Europe, for example, has been committed to addressing the issue of health inequality since the late 1970s (Whitehead 1992). In 1984 all thirty-two member states of the regional office unanimously agreed that 'by the year 2000, the actual differences in health status between countries and between groups within countries should be reduced by at least 25%, by improving the level of health of disadvantaged nations and groups' (Whitehead 1992, 429). In the 2000 edition of its annual statistical report, *The World Health Report 2000*, the WHO stated the importance of reporting on health inequality in order to determine how well the health system functions in each member country (Gakidou, Murray, and Frenk 2000; World Health Organization 2000a, 26). In 2005 the WHO established the Commission on the Social Determinants of Health, whose primary goal is to reduce health inequalities within and between countries (World Health Organization 2006). In addition, the World Bank is concerned about health inequality as part of its long-standing commitment to alleviate poverty (World Bank 2006).

Why are we interested in health inequality? Just as in any other scientific pursuit, we may simply be interested in describing the phenomenon, in this case how health is distributed among people. We may also wonder about the mechanism of health inequality. By studying the dynamics underlying an unequal health distribution, we may be able to improve our health.

Our interest in health inequality does not, however, always stop at describing and understanding unequal health distribution. Some health inequalities do not merely exist but also are of moral concern due to the value we place on health (Marchand, Wikler, and Landesman 1998; Peter and Evans 2001; Whitehead 1992). I believe this moral concern is what distinguishes health inequality as a topic, and moral concern about health inequality is the focus of this book. The moral or ethical dimension of health inequality is often termed health *inequity*, although no consensus on a precise definition of health inequity exists.

Moral concern for health inequality is sometimes explicitly stated. The WHO Regional Office for Europe, for example, has long expressed its commitment to the issue of health inequality as 'equity and health.' Moreover, a recent policy document of the British government, *Tackling Health Inequalities: A Programme for Action*, states: 'The reasons for these differences in health are, in many cases, avoidable and unjust – a consequence of differences in opportunity, in access to services, and material resources, as well as differences in the lifestyle choices of individuals' (UK Department of Health 2003, 6). But such explicit acknowledgments are rare. Rather, one must delve beneath the surface to discover the moral concerns underlying much health inequality analysis.

Consider, for example, a seemingly objective assessment of population health. A traditional indicator of the health of a population is the overall or average health. But the same average or overall level of health can be derived from different health distributions, as figure 1.1 shows. Population A, B, C, and D in figure 1.1 all have the same average number of life years. However, life years are more equally distributed across individuals in Population A than B (here, health distributions are plotted in much the same way that we often examine income inequality). Similarly, life years are more equally distributed between the poor and the rich in Population C than D. There is a growing consensus that in order to assess which population is healthier – Population A and B, or C and D, for example – one must be able to measure not only the average level of health across populations but inequalities in the level of health of individuals or groups within that population. In other words, it is increasingly accepted that a population is healthier when it has not only a higher overall or average level of health but also when it has less internal health inequality.

Although a consensus has yet to be reached as to among whom – individuals or groups – health inequality should be reduced (in other words, whether we should aim for Population A or C), these two goals are clearly endorsed in policy documents internationally (Public Health Agency of Canada 2002; U.S. Department of Health and Human Services 2000; Graham 2004; World Health Organization 2000a).

Making reduced health inequality a goal implies a judgment that greater health inequality is *worse* while smaller health inequality is *better*. Imagine that the inequality we were looking at in Population A, B, C, and D was the length of hair instead of the length of life. In this case, we might be curious about why the poor tend to have shorter hair than the rich, but we are unlikely to make a judgment that more equality in the length of hair is *better*. In the case of health inequality we are making a value judgment. Indeed, without this value judgment we do not know whether the health of a population improves when health inequality is reduced. The use of health inequality as a population health measure, therefore, presumes the moral implication of health inequality. *The World Health Report 2000* refers to the two goals as 'goodness' and 'fairness' rather than a higher overall or average health and a smaller health inequality (World Health Organization 2000a, 26).

Figure 1.1   The same average, different distributions

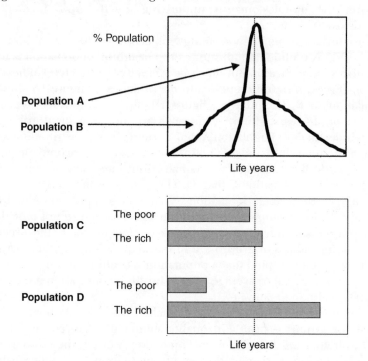

This choice of words explicitly acknowledges the ethical implication of health inequality.

This book is about measuring health inequality for moral reasons. More precisely, the focus of this book is the process of quantitatively describing health inequalities that concern us for moral reasons. Ultimately, the reason why we bother to measure health inequality relates to the value of collecting and reporting statistics. Accountability explains why we wish to, or even are obliged to, measure health inequality.[6]

Moral concern for health inequality implies social responsibility. Health inequality information collected in an appropriate way can tell us whether society is fulfilling this responsibility.

When our interest in health inequality is moral, the measurement strategy should reflect relevant moral concerns. Measuring health inequality in this sense is not an abstract, objective calculation detached from the real world and using alien-looking mathematical notations.

Rather, all the important questions that arise in thinking morally about health inequality are embedded in the construction and application of measurements of health inequality.

The interconnections between a moral concern with health inequality and health inequality measurement may not be immediately apparent. Let me clarify this point with examples. The concept of the 'right to health' is popular in international health circles (for example, Mann 1997). Advocates of this concept argue that health inequality is morally problematic because it reflects a violation of the right to health. The right to health resides in each person, just as each person has the right to vote. Thus, they would argue that health inequality be measured across individuals. To compare health inequality in Country A and B, supporters of the right to health might collect data and plot them on graphs as in figure 1.2a.[7] This figure suggests that health is distributed across individuals exactly the same way in Country A and B, and on would consequently conclude that Country A and B are the same in terms of health inequality.

Now imagine a social activist who has a different understanding of the moral implication of health inequality. She considers that systematic health inequality across social groups is a moral concern.[8] Such an investigator would not find the information in figure 1.2a particularly useful. Rather, she would need to look at how health is distributed across groups. She would compile different data and might plot them on graphs such as those in figure 1.2b. Despite the same overall health inequality across individuals, Country A and B are quite different with regard to the correlation between health and group affiliation. In Country A, members in cultural group 2 have fewer life years than members in cultural group 1. Group affiliation in Country B, on the other hand, does not determine one's health. According to the view that systematic health inequality across social groups is a moral concern, Country A is worse than Country B in terms of health inequality.

There is some evidence suggesting that this highly stylized example may not be entirely hypothetical. Around 1990, Japan and the United States had a similar degree of overall inequality in health-related quality of life (HRQL) across individuals measured by a summary index of inequality, the Gini coefficient (0.091 for the United States in 1990; 0.092 for Japan in 1989).[9] But inequality in HRQL by income was larger in the United States than in Japan. The difference in HRQL between the highest and lowest quintile of income earners was 0.12 in the United States and 0.03 in Japan. These differing results were obtained

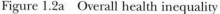

Figure 1.2a   Overall health inequality

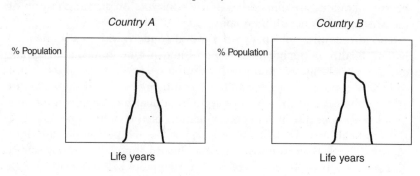

Figure 1.2b   Subpopulation health inequality

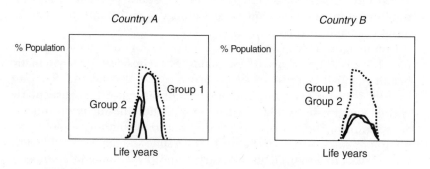

by different ways of measuring health inequality, each of which was based on different ways of thinking about the moral implications for health inequality. Thus, if one took the view of health inequality as a violation of the right to health, Japan and the United States were about the same. If, on the other hand, one adopted the view that systematic health inequality across social groups is a moral concern, then, the United States was worse than Japan.

1.2 Traditional and New Approaches

Given the importance of moral interests in health inequality, it is surprising that a comprehensive theoretical and analytical framework for measuring health inequality that acknowledges moral concerns has yet to be developed. Scholars in a variety of disciplines have a contribution to make to establish such a framework, but until recently such contributions have been minimal. Although philosophical arguments on equality are abundant, until recently philosophers have rarely addressed the issue of health in such discussions (Daniels 1985; Peter and Evans 2001). This is primarily due to the assumption that health is largely a natural good, whose distribution is beyond human control. The field of bioethics, the study of ethics in medicine, has concentrated primarily on individual relationships – for example, those between patients and physicians – and therefore generally lacks an interest in ethical issues at the population level.[10] Health care has often been a focus of moral consideration in these fields, but it is only recently that philosophers and bioethicists have directed their attention to health.[11] Health economists have long been interested in health care, but the moral implications of inequalities in health are relatively new to them.[12] Economists have made considerable progress in measuring income inequality, but they have shown little interest in exploring the analogy between measuring income inequality and measuring health inequality.

In the health field, measuring differences in health by socio-economic status (SES) has become the standard methodology of health inequality analysis. And researchers often assume that such health inequality has ethical implications. The rationale behind measuring differences in health by SES is, however, often intuitive. In developing a health inequality measurement for *The World Health Report 2000*, Murray, Gakidou, and Frenk challenged this traditional practice of measuring health inequality based on SES (1999). Although their proposal, on the whole, was not warmly received, it was a wake-up call, revealing that many more issues are at stake than is generally assumed. In the next section, I introduce in detail the practice of measuring health inequality by SES and the controversial proposal by Murray, Gakidou, and Frenk.

Health Inequality by Socio-economic Status

Traditionally, researchers have measured health inequality as differences in health by socio-economic status or social class. The relationship between SES and health is almost always that people with lower SES are on average sicker than people with higher SES. This relationship holds not only between the poor and the non-poor but also at every level of SES. This relationship can be vividly presented using the survival

Figure 1.3   Survival of women and children on the *Titanic*, by class

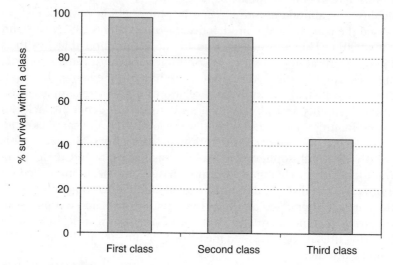

Source: Hall (1986).

rates on the S.S. *Titanic* by class (see figure 1.3). Survival rates were clearly affected by the class of the passage: the higher the class, the greater the chance of survival. If one substitutes the variable of life years for survival of the sinking of the *Titanic*, a similar pattern would emerge. This pattern is the so-called graded relationship between health and SES.

Questions as to when the graded relationship between health and SES first appeared in history, and whether health inequality by SES has been increasing or decreasing, do not have clear answers. They are disputed partly because no data, or no comparable data, are available. Researchers can measure health inequality by SES in many different ways, which makes its monitoring difficult. Still, Antonovsky (1967) speculates that the graded relationship between life expectancy and SES would not likely be significant when a whole society was struggling to survive. Based on historical analysis, he hypothesizes that differences in life expectancy by SES in Europe and North America were insignificant before the eighteenth century but grew in the nineteenth century. Since then, until around 1960, when Antonovsky conducted this analysis, differences in life expectancy by SES had narrowed. But when one looks at mortality rates instead of life expectancies by social class, another study suggests that health inequality by SES is increasing.[13]

Despite the lack of clarity of the historical trend, the persistence of health inequality by SES is undeniable. Most Western countries succeeded in providing health care to every citizen after the Second World War, and they naively and optimistically assumed that equal access to health care would produce equality in health outcome (Gunning-Schepers and Stronks 1999). Yet, differences in health by SES have persisted. At the dawn of the twenty-first century, evidence suggests that health inequality by SES is universal, both in developed and developing countries, and in countries with a universal health care system, including Scandinavian countries and Japan, whose social structure is often considered 'egalitarian.'[14]

What is remarkable about differences in health by SES is the consistency of the relationship. Differences in health by SES are observed both among men and women and across all ages, except possibly late old age. The differences are greater in middle to early old age (45–65 years old) than in earlier or later ages. The relationship between SES and health holds with various measurements of health, including mortality, morbidity (both curable and non-curable), self-perceived health, disability, and health-related quality of life. The only exceptions that have been reported are in the incidence of malignant melanoma and breast cancer: the incidence of these two diseases is greater among people of higher SES than among those of lower SES.[15]

The consistency in the relationship between health and SES is maintained despite the difficulty in measuring SES. Socio-economic status is considered a composite measure of three indicators that are 'interrelated but not fully overlapping': income, education, and occupational status (Adler et al. 1994). Studies do not use these indicators consistently: they sometimes measure only one or two of the items. Even when all three are measured, studies may use varying methods of collecting the information.

Researchers have proposed various hypotheses to explain the graded relationship between health and SES. Goldman's classification of these hypotheses is helpful: the relationship may be explained as (1) causal mechanisms, (2) selection or reverse causation, or (3) artifactual mechanisms (measurement error) (Goldman 2001). The category of selection or reverse causation is the hypothesis that illness forces people to move down the socio-economic ladder. Research has shown that this hypothesis is true to a small degree but does not explain all associations between health and socio-economic status (Wilkinson 1996, 59–60). Given the persistent observation of the relationship between health and SES, researchers have not seriously considered the third hypothesis.

Thus, the vast majority of research focuses on the first category, causal mechanisms. One can further classify hypotheses concerning causal mechanisms into two types, one focusing on *downstream causes*, and the other *upstream causes*. Downstream causes include material, behavioural, and psychological factors. Researchers argue that people with higher SES are on average healthier than those with lower SES because they possess more private and public resources, are 'quickest to acquire and act on information regarding health risks,' and/or have less stress and hostility, better coping skills, and a greater sense of control in their lives.[16]

Upstream causes are the factors that reflect the social structure. Wilkinson (1996), for example, argues that a hierarchical social structure in itself is the cause of differences in health by SES; Link and Phelan (1995) similarly claim SES as a fundamental cause of health inequality by SES. Income inequality is the upstream cause that has engendered the greatest debate. For this reason research in this area formed a distinct subfield within health inequality research in the 1990s.[17] Based on the observation that the greater the income inequality of a population, the sicker the overall population, the *relative income hypothesis* asserts that the health of an individual is determined not only by the absolute income of the individual but also by the income of others in the population. The validity of this hypothesis continues to be challenged both empirically (with questions about which countries to include in international analysis, how to define a population in within-country analysis, what factors should be controlled for, and how best to statistically model the relationship) and conceptually (whether the relationship between income inequality and population health indeed suggests the relative income hypothesis, and what mechanisms can explain the relative income hypothesis). Recent studies have revealed an 'American exceptionalism' (Ross, Tremblay, and Graham 2004; Wagstaff and van Doorslaer 2000): the relationship between greater income inequality and sicker population health appears to be evident primarily within the United States, and studies suggest that this relationship may exist only above a certain income inequality threshold. Whether the relative income hypothesis is true or false, the focus on income inequality in health inequality research has brought attention to community- or population-level determinants of health and has stimulated research into social cohesion and social capital.[18]

Whatever the true causal mechanisms, the observation of differences in health by SES prompts one of the most fundamental questions in health research, one reflected in the title of a 1994 book by Evans, Barer, and Marmor: Why are some people healthy and others not? The interest in differences in health by SES is, however, unlikely to be merely scientific. The ethical implications of the relative income hypothesis are obvious: as Daniels, Kennedy, and Kawachi provocatively claim in the title to their book, 'justice is good for our health' (2000). But even if income inequality was not the direct cause of differences in health by SES, the fact that health is differentiated by SES would strike many people as morally problematic. Part of the reason why studies on differences in health by SES have attracted so much attention is, Gunning-Schepers and Stronks argue, because 'the characteristics that define social inequalities between (sub) populations are at the very core of our social policies concerning distribution of wealth and power' (1999, 57).

The World Health Report 2000

The World Health Organization releases an annual world health report with a special theme and basic health statistics of its member countries. The theme for the year 2000 was the assessment of health systems. The task was led by then director Christopher Murray and then executive director Julio Frenk for Evidence and Information for Policy division (World Health Organization 2000a). *The World Health Report 2000* defined a health system as including 'all the activities whose primary purpose is to promote, restore or maintain health' (World Health Organization 2000a, 5) and distinguished two aspects of health system function: attainment, or what is achieved with respect to the three objectives of a health system; and performance, or how well a health system is functioning given the resources at hand. *The World Health Report 2000* suggested that each of these two aspects of health system function has three objectives: good health, responsiveness, and fair financial contribution. Importantly, *The World Health Report 2000* argued that the traditional focus on average or overall health and responsiveness is insufficient and that attention must also be paid to how health and responsiveness are distributed within a country. This ambitious concept produced the most controversial *World Health Report* in WHO history.[19]

One of the controversies surrounding the health system assessment in *The World Health Report 2000* is its proposed method for measuring health inequality (Gakidou, Murray, and Frenk 2000; Murray, Gakidou, and Frenk 1999).[20] Gakidou, Murray, and Frenk proposed to measure health inequality across individuals in much the same way as income inequality is measured. They defended their choice on two grounds. The first ground relates to measurement issues. They pointed out that using the individual as the unit of analysis allows international and longitudinal comparisons of health inequality more readily than if groups were the unit of analysis. The second ground concerns the moral stand implied by the choice of the unit of analysis. Researchers have often assumed that there is a moral implication to measuring health inequality by groups. Gakidou, Murray, and Frenk asserted that health inequality across individuals is also of moral concern. One could infer that they questioned why the normative position implied by addressing health inequality across groups should take precedence over other normative positions.

The proposal by Gakidou, Murray, and Frenk has received fierce criticism from researchers and policy-makers in the field of health inequality.[21] Most of the criticism attacked the moral implications of the unit of analysis rather than measurement issues. This fact itself is telling about the importance of moral issues in seemingly morally neutral measurement practice. Advocates of the group approach, especially those who equate health inequality with differences in health by SES, do not think that health inequality across individuals is morally significant. Furthermore, without any group information, they do not think that health inequality across individuals provides any guidance as to how to reduce health inequality.

In chapters 2 and 3, I evaluate the claims and justifications made by Gakidou, Murray, and Frenk and their opponents. Even if Gakidou, Murray, and Frenk were wrong in everything they said about the unit of analysis in measurement of health inequality (which is not my view), one cannot deny that they initiated a stimulating discussion. Advocates of the traditional approach can no longer rest on tradition; they must defend their approach. Why, for example, is focusing on the health of the poor of greater moral concern than focusing on the health of the sick? The unit of analysis is but one issue that Gakidou, Murray, and Frenk raise in health inequality measurement. One must acknowledge that they began an important discussion on what aspects of health we should measure and in what way for what reasons. Even though their effort is still in its infancy, and I myself am among its critics, I believe that their measurement of health inequality is the most comprehensive to date. An exciting era of measuring health inequality to reflect moral concerns has just began.

1.3 The Aim and the Plan

This book responds to the growing interest in and need for health inequality measurement to reflect moral concerns. To that end, it aims to build a theoretical and analytical framework for measuring health inequality. This requires a philosophical investigation of the value we place on health and its distribution, as well as an examination of quantitative methodologies that transform philosophical concepts into useful tools for policy-making.

The uniqueness of this project lies in the marriage of philosophy and quantitative methodologies. The general goal of this book is to establish a framework for measuring health inequality where important moral and quantitative questions are critically reviewed and analysed. The framework is pluralistic. It is not my intention to defend one particular measurement based on a certain normative position. I hope this book will be useful to all of those, from academics to policy-makers, who are concerned about the moral implications of health inequality in populations of various types and sizes.

Measuring health inequality to reflect moral concerns is a uniquely multidisciplinary endeavour. A book on such a topic can be exciting but is also demanding. It asks readers to appreciate various methods of communication: by words, numbers, diagrams, tables, and figures. It urges readers to build bridges between their own discipline and others. Although my goal was to make the discussion as accessible as possible, some sections may prove challenging to some readers. Difficulty in understanding every part of this book comes inevitably from the multidisciplinary nature of the topic. Unsatisfactory understanding of some parts should only encourage readers to work on the topic of measuring health inequality within multidisciplinary teams.

This book consists of two parts. Part 1 is conceptual: in it I develop a framework for measuring health inequality that acknowledges moral concerns. Part 2 is empirical: there I present case studies to show exactly how empirical research can be conducted using this framework.

Part 1 comprises three chapters. They correspond to three steps involved in measuring health inequality to reflect moral concerns: (1) defining which health distributions are inequitable, (2) deciding on measurement strategies to operationalize a chosen concept of equity,

Figure 1.4   Three steps for measuring health inequality
for moral concerns

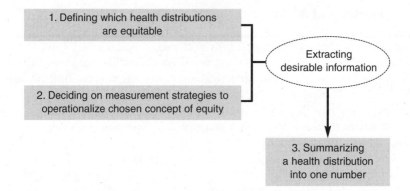

and (3) summarizing a health distribution into one number, or quantifying health inequality information (figure 1.4).[22] In the first two steps,
the desirable information is extracted from the health distribution. In
the last step, the desirable information is condensed in a form that is easy
to communicate. All three steps ask distinct questions. After clarifying
the terminology used in this project and providing preliminary discussion on various reasons why we might be ethically interested in health
distribution, I examine these three steps in order in these chapters.

For many readers chapter 4 will be the most demanding in the book.
It is an intricate interchange between philosophy and numbers; this is
the chapter that speaks most to the multidisciplinary nature of measuring health inequality. I limit mathematical notation as much as possible,
in order to make this material as accessible as possible. For those who
wish to avoid technical issues altogether, I suggest skipping section 4.4.

In part 2 (chapters 5 and 6) I present empirical analyses that apply a
variety of moral perspectives on health inequality derived from part 1.
The data for these case studies are from the 1990 and 1995 U.S.
National Health Interview Survey. I use these same data to determine,
from a number of different moral perspectives, whether health equity
improved in the United States between 1990 and 1995. The primary
objective of part 2 is to show the connection between the conceptual
and empirical analyses of health inequality. Every measurement decision I make in the empirical analyses in part 2 derives from the discussions in part 1.

Parts 1 and part 2 are integral components for measuring health inequality to reflect moral concerns. For this reason, I encourage even readers with little quantitative training to read part 2. Such readers might approach part 2 as if they were part of a multidisciplinary team measuring health inequality reflecting moral concern and were listening to a colleague with quantitative training explain how the concept they developed together was used in the actual measurement practice. I attempt to explain quantitative methods in ordinary language. Nonetheless, should readers wish to avoid quantitative materials altogether, I suggest they read only sections 5.1 and 5.3 in Chapter 5 and section 6.2 Chapter 6. I encourage readers with a quantitative orientation to read the appendices for precise definitions and for further exploration of the quantitative methodologies used.

In concluding the book, chapter 7 provides a summary of each chapter and identifies future work.

1.4 Terminology

Different researchers have used the term 'health inequality' in different ways, and there are numerous other terms that appear to suggest similar meanings or whose concepts closely relate to the meaning of health inequality.[23] Such words include, but are not limited to, difference, disparity, heterogeneity, inequity, and injustice. There is also the problem of the antonym – philosophers discuss equality, while economists discuss inequality (Temkin 1993, 7).

Figure 1.5 illustrates the operational classification of terminologies that I use for this book. *Health distribution* is a way in which health is spread among the parties of interest in a population of concern. These parties can be individuals or groups of individuals, and I sometimes refer to a population as a society. *Health equality* is the health distribution in which health is spread equally to every party in a population of concern, and *health inequality* is all health distributions that are otherwise. Reducing health inequality is the same as increasing health equality. Despite the different connotation of each word, I assume that such terms as difference, disparity,[24] and heterogeneity in health have the same meaning as health inequality. Some health distributions are of moral concern, and the ethical dimension of health distribution is *health inequity*. Note that not only health inequality but also health equality could cause moral concerns.[25] Chapter 2 aims to introduce diverse views about health inequity.

Figure 1.5   Terminology

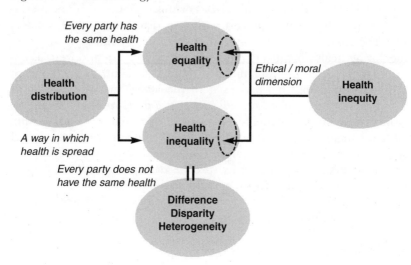

Inequitable health distribution implies social responsibility. The health inequity perspectives I look at in this book are those based on concerns for justice: these perspectives identify which health distributions society ought to be morally concerned about and act upon.

1.5 Preliminary Discussion: Why Are We Morally Interested in Health Distribution?

In any research activity, different interests lead to different research strategies. The analysis of health distribution is no exception. Researchers and policy-makers, however, do not always explicitly communicate why they are interested in health distribution, and, if their interests relate to moral concerns, what those concerns are. Along with data availability and technical issues regarding quantitative analysis, clarification of one's exact interest in health distribution should play an important role in opting for a certain measurement strategy. Preliminary to a discussion of this book, in this section I look at different types of moral concerns for health distribution.

In classifying diverse ethical concerns regarding health distribution, it is useful to examine whether our interest in health distribution is instrumental for realizing other ideals. We might be concerned about health distribution because it affects other ethical ideals that we care about most. The *utilitarian* perspective is one of the examples of such distribution-insensitive ethical concerns for health distribution (that is, that ethical concerns apply regardless of the distribution). Utilitarians, thinking about the health of a population, would wish the highest average health of the population possible, irrespective of how health is distributed within a population. Marchand, Wikler, and Landesman (1998) point out that *The Black Report* (Black et al. 1992), which is usually considered to show a commitment to equal health distribution, actually shares a utilitarian perspective.

As an argument for reducing health inequality, Woodward and Kawachi introduce the view that '[health] inequalities affect everyone' (2000, 923). They state, for example, that 'some types of health inequalities have obvious spillover effects on the rest of society, for example, the spread of infectious diseases, the consequences of alcohol and drug misuse, or the occurrence of violence and crime' (2000, 923). This view is a variant of the utilitarian perspective as it posits that some health inequalities are problematic because they prevent people in the population from reaching their potential for better health or general well-being.

We might, on the other hand, be interested in health distribution because of its intrinsic moral significance. Unlike the utilitarians, egalitarians would be concerned primarily about how health is distributed within a population regardless of its relationship to the population's overall level of health or well-being.[26] We may eventually need to balance the concern for health equity with other goals of population health. But our interest in health equity is not instrumental in realizing other ideals.

It is straightforward for researchers to say that they are interested in describing how health is spread within a population and investigating the mechanisms of the distribution. Similarly, it is clear what is meant if researchers say they are concerned about health distribution because it greatly influences the population health goal that they believe to be the most important. When researchers say, however, that they are morally concerned about health distribution without reference to other population health goals, the meaning is less clear. Why might health distribution present moral questions? There are at least three reasons: (a) health is a special good and its distribution is of moral importance, (b) health equity plays an important role in the general pursuit of justice, and (c) health inequality is an indicator of general social justice.[27] These three reasons loosely form a basis of different perspectives on health equity that I will look at in the next chapter.

Health as a Special Good

Some scholars argue that the reason for our moral concern with health inequality is that health is a special good (S. Anand 2002; Culyer 2001). Health is, first and foremost, an important component of welfare or well-being. Health contributes to our overall happiness and satisfaction and, generally speaking, helps us feel comfortable about ourselves. Anand believes that this intrinsic value of health distinguishes it from other important goods such as income, whose value is primarily instrumental (S. Anand 2002, 485). Furthermore, health is a multi-purpose resource necessary and useful for any conception of a good life. While there are other important resources – for example, income and education – health can be seen as the most fundamental resource of all. Income and education would be of no value if we were dead. Woodward and Kawachi write that 'poor health is one of the most important causes of restricted opportunity and limited personal freedom' (2000, 6). Writing in the eighteenth century, Thomas Jefferson went further: 'Without health there is no happiness.'[28] 'Human flourishing' is closely tied to health; consequently, some see health as a special good (Culyer 2001, 281). And, if they are correct, is it not inevitable that we pay particular attention to health equity? Certainly, according to Jefferson, who claimed that 'an attention to health, then, should take place of every other object.'

This perspective focuses on health equity independently from equities in other important goods. A strong justification has yet to be made as to whether focusing solely on health is conceptually and tactically appealing, but this view is fairly prevalent in the health sciences literature (for example, Culyer and Wagstaff 1993; Gakidou, Murray, and Frenk 2000). Tobin refers to the position that focuses on equity in a specific sphere as *specific egalitarianism*, while Peter and Evans refer to it as the *direct approach* (Peter 2001; Peter and Evans 2001; Tobin 1970).

Health Equity and the Pursuit of Justice

Others, especially philosophers, are a little cautious about claiming special status for health. Rather, they are more likely to examine the concept of equality in general. Philosophy has a long tradition of discussing equality and justice,[29] and its arguments – at least within contemporary Western philosophy – share a fundamental premise: we ought to respect all persons equally (Gosepath 2001; Hausman, forthcoming). Different theories are born from disagreement about exactly what we should seek to equalize.

In philosophical discussions of equality, a person is understood as being born with certain internal characteristics – for example, particular abilities and personality. Depending on where individuals are born, they receive different external resources – for example, a specific family setting or social status. These internal characteristics and external resources together predict an individual's potential for the future. In other words, they determine the degree of freedom that person enjoys (Amartya Sen [1992] uses the term *capabilities* to refer to this relative degree of freedom). Making personal choices and facing random chance events, individuals realize outcomes or welfare. Philosophers have directed their attention to different focal points in this understanding of a person, believing that equality of the chosen focal point is the best way to express equal moral respect for all persons. Well-theorized focal points include equality in resources, welfare, opportunities for welfare, and capabilities.[30]

Whatever the theoretical focal point, philosophers have rarely discussed health. In their understanding, health is primarily a natural good, whose distribution is beyond human control. Health care has often been a focus of moral consideration in these arguments, but it is only recently that some philosophers have begun to perceive health primarily as a social good (Marchand, Wikler, and Landesman 1998; Peter and Evans 2001), and have reflected upon the broad understanding of determinants of population health, including social and physical environment, genetic endowment, individual behavioural and biological responses, and health care (Evans and Stoddart 1990). Some scholars have begun to think that health might be included in the list of goods whose distribution is of moral interest. That is, health might be considered to be a resource in the resourcist view, one component of welfare in the welfarist view, and the like.[31] If we perceive health as a good whose distribution is of moral interest, then logically we are morally concerned about health distribution, because seeking health equity is a part of the general pursuit of equality or justice. Peter and Evans call this position the *indirect approach* (Peter 2001; Peter and Evans 2001).

Like the specific egalitarian, those who regard health as a good whose distribution is of moral interest agree that health is special but only to the degree that it should be included in the proper space of egalitarian concern. To them, unlike the specific egalitarian, health does not automatically call for special attention over other goods. Its importance must be weighed against these other goods. If we concluded that health was only as special as other important goods, we would find our moral concerns for health in its relation to other goods. Health distribution in

~~this view would have to be measured in relation to distributions of other~~ goods. Others might argue that health has a particular moral significance even among other important goods, just as we frequently regard political liberty as a special good within the scope of equality. Still others might argue that health is only as special as other important goods but might present a practical justification for why we pay special attention to health – for example, that health can be treated as an indicator of the entire set of important goods.

With reference to measurement, those who prefer the indirect approach, but in one way or another justify extracting health from other equity considerations, would be indistinguishable from the specific egalitarian: both of them would measure only health. Walzer (1983) proposes a view of 'complex equality,' in which he argues that there are a number of spheres of justice in our lives and that each sphere is governed by a distinctive set of rules. Such a set of rules is determined by characteristics of the sphere in question and specific conditions of the society within which the sphere takes shape. We might wish to include health as a sphere in Walzer's complex equality. The starting point is then a general pursuit of justice, yet, at the measurement level, we could reasonably be concerned only about health equity.

Health Inequality as an Indicator of General Social Justice

The two views introduced above derive their interest in the distribution of health from its moral significance. However, we might be morally concerned about health distribution not so much because of the value of health in itself but rather because of its relationships to other goods. Multiple factors, including the distribution of commodities and the general functioning of a society, determine health outcomes and health inequality. Health inequality can thus be regarded as an indicator of general social justice. In the classification by Peter and Evans (Peter 2001; Peter and Evans 2001), this is still an indirect approach, as health equity is considered within a larger framework of social justice. But the direction of interests runs from health to social justice.

These three reasons why we might ethically be interested in health distribution can be developed from a variety of perspectives, which make different judgments on exactly which health distributions are ethically problematic. The next chapter introduces these different perspectives on health equity.

PART ONE

Framework

2 Which Health Distributions Are Inequitable?

2.1 Introduction

In this chapter I introduce a variety of egalitarian perspectives on health equity. For the purpose of this book 'egalitarianism' means that we are morally concerned about health distribution itself, rather than treating it as instrument for realizing other ideals of population health. So constrained, this chapter asks: which health distributions are inequitable?

To investigate this question, we must examine how health might fit within a general philosophical discussion of equality.[1] Philosophers have argued over equality for thousands years, producing countless perspectives, while never completely agreeing with each other. Tackled squarely, my task is insurmountable. I therefore limit myself to the introduction of the different perspectives on health equity already proposed, most often only intuitively, in the health sciences literature, classifying them, and giving a flavour of how they might be associated with general philosophical discussions of equality. If one wants to know more about genuine philosophical arguments, there are abundant philosophical articles. What health researchers most want to know is what terms like 'health equity' or 'justice' really mean in the health sciences literature. Can philosophy help explain them a bit more? This chapter aims to do just that.

As a first step, I categorize perspectives on health equity into two groups: equity as equality in health, and health inequality as an indicator of social justice. Perspectives in the first group are more popular than the second, and I accordingly give more attention to these perspectives. I start by introducing what is presumably the most straightforward idea of strict equality in health outcome and argue why it does not provide an attractive account of health equity. I then discuss different views that relax such strictness in two ways, by cause and by level. After reviewing both groups of equity perspectives, I revisit the three egalitarian reasons to be interested in health distribution discussed in the introduction and look at how they connect to different perspectives on health equity introduced in this chapter.

2.2 Equity as Equality in Health

Strict Equality of Health Outcome

If one held the view that health is to some degree special, equality of health outcome might appear to be the most straightforward criterion for health equity. This sentiment is sometimes expressed in the health sciences literature; for example, Culyer states:

> An equitable health care policy should seek to reduce the inequality in health (life expectation, self-reported morbidity, quality of life in terms of personal and social functioning) at every stage of the life-cycle. Such policy must meet needs, but in the proportion to the 'distance' each individual is from the population average. Constraints may be desirable, some of which might be based on merit arguments. Moreover, it is probably not ethical to seek greater equality of health by reducing the health of the already relatively healthy. There may be compromises between the ethical desiderata of equity and efficiency in cases where egalitarian policies could reduce the variance of health only by causing total health to deteriorate. (2001, 281)

In essence, Culyer says that we should aim primarily for strict equality of health outcome (in his case, at the population's average health level) with some appropriate adjustments.

Can this intuitive appeal to the view of strict equality of health outcome be in any way justified? Let us first be clear about what strict equality of health outcome means. Note that Culyer's support for strict equality of health outcome is conditional upon not harming the healthy. Does this condition weaken his commitment to egalitarianism? For someone to be an egalitarian, should she not always favour equality even at the expense of harming the healthy? A common claim that egalitarians always favour equality even when it is achieved by pulling the better-off down is called the levelling-down objection. Some scholars consider this objection as a fatal problem of egalitarianism and suggest that rather than egalitarian views we support the priority (Parfit 1991) or extended humanitarian (Temkin 1993, chap. 9) view, where we give priority to the worst-off over the better-off (Arneson 2002, sec. 5.2). Prioritarians argue that what is morally problematic in inequality is not that someone fares worse than others but that the worst-off have not achieved the level that they could have achieved. As long as policy to reduce inequality improved the condition of the worst-off, prioritarians would support it. The levelling-down objection in the health context is, for example, that prioritarians would object to health equality achieved by genocide in a population because genocide does not improve the health of the worst-off, while egalitarians would still prefer health equality even in this case.

Broome (n.d.), Fleurbaey (n.d. a), and Hausman (n.d. a) disagree with the old claim that levelling-down situations separate prioritarians and egalitarians, although they diverge as to whether the distinction between prioritarians and egalitarians is meaningful. Hausman distinguishes egalitarians and narrower 'egalitarians' (Hausman n.d. a). He defines egalitarians as 'those who favour lessening inequalities, because of their commitment to moral principles linked to distribution' (n.d. a, 2) and 'egalitarians' as 'those who place an intrinsic value on equality of distribution, regardless of its contribution to other goals' (n.d., 1). 'Egalitarians' can value other goals such as efficiency in addition to equity, and may eventually balance equity and other goals, *all things considered*. But when judging which distribution is better *in terms of equity*, 'egalitarians' always prefer equality over inequality. Egalitarians may not; they do not simply prefer equality to any inequalities because judgment on which distribution is better in terms of equity depends on why we care about certain distributions. In other words, the levelling-down objection only applies to 'egalitarians,' but not to egalitarians. Broome, Fleurbaey, and Hausman argue that it is hard to find situations where prioritarians and egalitarians disagree about which distribution is better in terms of equity,[2] and Fleurbaey and Hausman continue that differences between them are reasons for the judgment and measurement approaches.[3]

I share the broad definition of egalitarians. Understanding egalitarianism in the broad sense, the levelling-down objection is not a threat to egalitarianism, and Culyer's view of strict equality of health outcomes conditional upon not harming the healthy is an egalitarian perspective.

Now let us go back to our question: can the intuitive appeal to the view of strict equality of health outcome, as expressed by Culyer, be in any way justified? One possibility is to perceive health as a good resembling political liberty. If we characterize health in such a way, strict equality of health outcome might be defended as strict equality of political liberty. This line of argument can be developed along with John Rawls's theory of justice as fairness (1971), one of the most influential ideas of the twentieth century. Let us here briefly review Rawls's theory of justice as fairness.

Rawls suggests that we begin our consideration behind a 'veil of ignorance,' where people are assumed to lack knowledge of who they are, including their personalities, socio-economic positions, and beliefs, while at the same time maintaining general understanding of the world. In this strange condition, Rawls's 'original position,' they must adopt basic rules of the society in which they live. Rawls then asks what kind of rules they might agree upon. Rawls suggests two such rules: 'first, each person is to have an equal right to the most extensive basic liberty compatible with a similar liberty for others, and second, social and economic inequalities are to be arranged so that they are both (a) reasonably expected to be to everyone's advantage, and (b) attached to positions and offices open to all' (1971, 60). Note that these two principles have different references as to among whom equality should be sought. The first principle is concerned with the equal provision of political liberty to each person, while the second principle seeks socioeconomic equality among 'representative persons holding the various social positions, or offices, or whatever, established by the basic structure' (1971, 64). Rawls calls the second rule the *difference principle*, and it is also frequently referred to as the *maxmin* – maximizing the minimum – *principle*. These two rules are in the 'lexicographical [or as Rawls abbreviates, lexical] order,' meaning that the first must be met before the second.

Rawls says that there are such things as primary goods that 'normally have a use whatever a person's rational plan of life,' and that therefore 'every rational man is presumed to want' (1971, 62). He thinks that distributions of some primary goods, for example, liberty and opportunity, income and wealth, offices, and the bases of self-respect, are influenced by the basic structure of society in an important way and calls them social primary goods. He goes on to suggest that there is another type of primary goods whose 'possession is influenced by the basic structure, [but] they are not directly under its control' (1971, 62). He calls these natural primary goods and lists such goods as health and vigour, intelligence and imagination as examples. The theory of justice that Rawls proposes is concerned about the distribution of social primary goods, but not natural primary goods. Health is thus outside the consideration of his framework.

Some philosophers challenge this point and examine the possibility of incorporating health in the Rawlsian framework (Daniels 1985; Daniels, Kennedy, and Kawachi 2000, 2004; Peter 2001). To expand Rawls's theory of justice, a decision must first be made as to whether health can be or should be included in the list of social primary goods. If so, one then must ask which of the two principles should govern the distribution of health, the principle applied to the basic liberty goods or the difference principle. As we discussed in the introduction, given the central role of health in human flourishing, one might believe that it is closer to political liberty rather than to such social primary goods as income and wealth. If this could be justified, then health distribution should be governed in a way similar to political liberty, that is, on the basis of strict equality to each person. One might instead think that health is an all-purpose resource like income and wealth and that its distribution among representative persons of the social hierarchy should be governed by the difference principle. We will discuss this view further below in the section on inequity as health inequality by socio-economic status.

Strict equality in health outcome, understood literally, is obviously not an attractive perspective on health equity. First, there is a problem of choice. Multiple factors determine health outcomes, and one of them is personal health behaviour. Under serious scrutiny, perfectly free-willed, informed health behaviour may scarcely exist, but let us assume that there is such behaviour. While we hope and encourage people to seek a healthy lifestyle, in practice compulsion is rare. We do have, for example, the seat belt law and labour standards acts, but we do not force people to engage in certain hours of exercise a week or to quit smoking. Nor do we punish them for the consequences of their irresponsible health behaviours. Access to health care does not discriminate against people on the ground of their health behaviours, though it often does so in the United States for such factors as the ability to pay (Wikler 1987). Why are we tolerant of irresponsible health behaviours? We are because we value personal choice and accept that people make trade-offs between health and other goods in their lives. This suggests that health may be a good resembling, but not exactly like, political liberty, which is in principle understood as untradable.

Another notable difference between political liberty and health is cost. For simplicity, let us assume that political liberty is a vote. Apart from the administrative cost to ensure equality, it costs almost nothing to distribute a strictly equal vote to each person, that is, one vote to one person. In contrast, society could bankrupt itself if it tried to provide strictly equal health to everyone.[4] In every society there would always be the sick whose health we just cannot improve, even with all medical care currently available. And there is a paradox of health production: 'a society which spends so much on health care that it cannot or will not spend adequately on other health enhancing activities may actually be *reducing* the health of its population though increased health spending' (Evans and Stoddart 1990, 1360, original emphasis).

The problem of choice not only raises the issue of freedom but also that of responsibility. Recall that we are here talking about what kind of health distributions society ought to be concerned about and act upon. Should society be responsible for health outcomes caused by perfectly free-willed, informed risk-taking health behaviour, say, as in someone becoming a quadriplegic due to an accident while bungee jumping? With limited resources it might be reasonable to say that individuals rather than society should be at least to some degree responsible for the reduction of health due to free, informed, risky health behaviour.

Another problem with a strict equality of health outcome is related to chance. Rawls is right in saying that the distribution of health is not directly under social control – there are always unfortunate health outcomes beyond human control. While we may reasonably feel sorry for a baby born with an incurable birth defect, with no clear indication of why it happened we may be hesitant to hold society fully responsible.

Health may be special, but not so special as to require a strict equality of health outcome. The strictness must be relaxed in some way or another for this view to be plausible.

Focusing on Cause

From the preceding discussion, it is obvious that strict equality in health outcome is unlikely to be an attractive perspective on health equity. In fact, popular accounts of health equity relax the strictness of the view of strict equality in health outcome in one way or another. The most common way to do so is to think about health determinants and define health inequalities caused by certain determinants as health inequity. This view is so predominant that many health researchers seem to think that health equity cannot be defined without information on health determinants. Whitehead, for example, says: 'The term "inequity" has a moral and ethical dimension. It refers to differences which are *unnecessary* and *avoidable*, but in addition are considered *unfair and unjust*. So, in order to describe a certain situation as inequitable the *cause* has to be examined and *judged* to be unfair in the *context* of what is going on in the rest of society' (1992, 431, original emphasis). Later I will introduce the view that incorporating the causal information is not the only way to define health equity, but here we will look at different perspectives proposed under this popular category. Before introducing specific perspectives, I will first set forth a general framework for thinking about health determinants in the moral investigation of the health distribution. I will then turn to three perspectives, each of which pays attention to health inequalities caused by different factors.

HEALTH DETERMINANTS IN MORAL INVESTIGATION
OF HEALTH DISTRIBUTION

Multiple factors determine health. To investigate the moral relevance of health distributions, let us start by categorizing health determinants into three groups: (I) responsibility of society (social arrangement), (II) choice, and (III) nobody's fault, that is, neither social nor individual responsibility. This categorization is surely oversimplified. Yet let us assume that these three categories can be identified when our conceptual analysis of human behaviour and corresponding empirical methodology become sufficiently sophisticated. Table 2.1 presents examples of variables for each category. Recent empirical health determinant studies have shown that variables at the individual as well as community levels are important predictors of health (for example, Robert and House 2000). Accordingly, examples in table 2.1 are divided into the individual and community level variables. To highlight the characteristic of each category, I will first introduce the three categories as if each of them existed independently. Interactions between them will then enter into the consideration so our discussion becomes realistic.

Health determinants categorized under Group I, for example, are income, education, and access to health care at the individual level. These are factors whose distribution is largely determined by social arrangements. They include proxies for socio-economic status or social class.

Group II health determinants are personal and community choices for healthy life. Such lifestyle factors as drinking, exercise, and diet, and

Table 2.1
Classification of health determinants for moral investigation

Group	Characteristic	Variable example	
		Individual level	Community level
I	Responsibility of society	Income, education, access to health care	% poverty in community, safe water supply, safety legislation, design of physical environment
II	Choice	Lifestyle (e.g., drinking), risky leisure activity	
III	Nobody's fault	Sex, age, chance (accident)	War, famine, epidemic

a risky leisure activity such as skydiving are examples at the individual level. Community level determinants in the social responsibility and choice categories are closely related to each other, as a community choice is what a community decides to do (or not to do) as a collective will. Such variables as the percentage of people below the poverty level in a community, safe water supply, safety legislation, and design of the physical environment can be understood in either of these categories.

Group III health determinants are ones that we cannot do anything about. Roughly speaking, at the individual level this category includes chance and biological variations. Chance determinants, also termed 'brute luck' in the philosophy literature, are, for example, such random misfortunes as being hit by lightning. Biological determinants are, for example, age and sex. Because all determinants of health eventually affect the biological process of a human body, it might sound a little confusing to acknowledge such a category as biological variations. But these factors are direct characteristics that all individuals of the human species possess, that is, all human beings are either male or female and everyone gets one year older every year. In this sense, I believe that these specific biological determinants can stand as a conceptually distinct category. We can think of war, famine, and epidemics as examples of community-level variables in this category. Note that as technology improves some effects of the Group III determinants at both levels can become controllable.

Genetics is also an example of a Group III health determinant, and it interestingly possesses both characteristics of chance and biology. A gene has more of the chance characteristic when its distribution (or the distribution of its outcome) is unequal, our knowledge about it is limited, or it interacts greatly with the environment. With a few exceptions, given the current knowledge of genetics, genes are perhaps best characterized as chance determinants. Even when the field of genetics further develops, many genes will still be best understood as having more of the characteristic of chance than biology. How a gene affects our health, as with many other types of determinants, is of course a biological process. But 'biology' in our usage here means a shared human experience as characterized by age and sex. We must recognize also the internal feature of genetics as a chance determinant. Chance acquisition happens at the very beginning of life for genetics,[5] while it usually takes place in later life for such other chance events as being hit by lightning. This difference becomes important when we look closely at health in chapter 3.

Obviously, health determinants rarely exist in a way that can clearly fit into one of the three categories. Interactions between these three categories are apparent. Sex, for example, is a biological variation, but at the same time it is more than biology; its meaning is also socially shaped and interpreted. Socially shaped characteristics based on biological sex are referred to as gender. Both gender and sex determine our health. The observation, for example, that women tend to live longer than men can be regarded as a biological effect of sex.[6] On the other hand, epidemiological data suggesting that men have higher violence-related mortality rates than women may be regarded as reflecting different social norms that the society imposes on men, that is, gender. Acknowledging biological and social aspects of sex, sex is an interaction between Group III, nobody's fault, and Group I, social responsibility.

Similarly, the chance of being shot is a good example of interaction between Group I, social arrangement, and Group III, nobody's fault determinants. While the probability of being shot with a firearm is random in some cases, health statistics suggest that this may not actually be so: the poor and people living in poor neighbourhoods have a higher probability of being shot. Consider another example: what if there is a genetic disease whose distribution is random but treatment for which is provided more favourably to the rich than the poor?

Interaction between Group I, social responsibility, and Group III, nobody's fault determinants, is well known. Empirical studies, for example, suggest that personal choice for healthy behaviour is often correlated with socio-economic factors. Although there is disagreement as to degree, it is generally accepted in the health research community that health behaviours are partly socially determined.

Furthermore, Group II, choice, and Group III, nobody's fault, determinants also interact. Not all smokers develop lung cancer, perhaps with the help of protective biological mechanisms that we cannot yet identify, or simply by chance. A minority of unlucky bungee jumpers die, but most of them survive. Individuals make choices, but the consequences of these choices are not always under their control.

Variables at the community level are no exception to such interactions. For example, being born at a specific time and location where war, famine, or epidemic exist is itself a random event we can do nothing about. But we can easily imagine that such misfortune may well devastate people to different degrees according to their social strata. Can we then still say that the effects of disaster on health are entirely nobody's fault? Social structure is to some degree responsible for the unequal share of burdens.

Given so many interactions between the three categories, one might wonder whether the three categories in table 2.1 really exist as distinctive groups. This suspicion can be found, for example, in the question of whether there is such a thing as social responsibility or individual choice. People in a variety of fields, including health, have discussed this question for a number of years,[7] and this is perhaps one of the most fundamental issues in any analysis of human behaviour. Reflecting upon the large majority of empirical analyses of health inequality by socioeconomic status (SES), I listed in table 2.1 income and education as examples of health determinants whose distributions are a social responsibility. Yet there is no doubt that each individual to some degree makes decisions on how much money she earns and how much education she invests for herself. As Le Grand says, a 'complete denial of free will' touches on the fundamental assumption in health policy (1991, 117), and indeed on our understanding of human beings. One would then wonder about a reasonable middle ground: how much of a personal choice is a free, voluntary choice, and how much is socially determined? A clear answer to this question is yet to be discovered. Isaiah Berlin's defence of freedom in individual decision making, for example, candidly expresses the complexity of this question:

> When everything has been said in favor of attributing responsibility for character and action to natural and institutional causes; when everything possible has been done to correct blind or over-simple interpretations of

conduct which fix too much responsibility on individuals and their free acts; when in fact there is strong evidence to show that it was difficult or impossible for men to do otherwise than they did, given their material environment or education or the influence upon them of various 'social pressures'; when every relevant psychological and sociological considera- tion has been taken into account, every impersonal factor given due weight after all these severities, we continue to praise and to blame. (1969, 96)

It is one thing to recognize the complexity of the question at the con- ceptual level. But this does not stop empirical investigation of health equity. Reasonable assumptions must be sought, but how? John Roemer suggests one way how we might distinguish social responsibility and per- sonal choice (Roemer et al. 1995). Roemer categorizes human actions in two groups: one is caused by circumstances beyond individual control, and the other individual autonomous choices. He advocates equality of opportunity that equalizes outcomes caused by factors beyond individual control but permits unequal outcomes caused by individual autonomous choices. He shows us with examples how we might decide which parts of human actions are due to autonomous choices or factors beyond individual control. Although his idea ulti- mately fails to provide a solution, it seems worth considering as a possi- ble step forward in searching for a measurement strategy.

Let us take his example of smoking. Roemer invites us to imagine a White, female college professor who has smoked eight years in her life, and a Black, male steelworker who has smoked thirty years in his life. The median period of smoking for such people as the college professor, that is, White, female college professors, is eight years, while for people like Black, male steelworkers it is thirty years. While in absolute numbers the college professor smoked twenty-two years less than the steelworker, Roemer argues that their smoking experiences should be considered the same if we adjust for the factor of how hard it was to make the choice not to smoke in each situation. If this was a question of com- pensation for medical care for lung cancer, Roemer continues, a society should compensate people of the college professor's 'type' who smoked for less than eight years and people of the steelworker's 'type' who smoked for less than thirty years.

Roemer's intuitively appealing idea has been criticized in various ways. For example, what does it really mean to be responsible for making autonomous choices? Scanlon argues that 'even though [people] *are* responsible for making certain choices (they are, for example, properly criticized for so doing), we ought to help them nonetheless' (Roemer et al. 1995, original emphasis). In addition, how can we possibly implement Roemer's idea given that human character- istics can be divided into the countless number of 'types'? How can we collect all necessary information? Furthermore, even if we agreed on a certain limited number of reasonable 'types,' an oversight agency is nec- essary to implement Roemer's idea. Who can play that role? Will we be comfortable with such an oversight agency? Is it not arrogant even to begin to think that we can calculate all causation of life events?

Should we wish to apply Roemer's idea to health inequality measure- ment, the most challenging obstacle among the criticisms would be impracticality. An immediate difficulty is that there are too many ways to categorize people. Roemer's smoking example is characterized by sex, race, and occupation, but are these 'types' sufficient to describe dif- ferent environments for smoking? Although this is a difficult question, it is not insurmountable. Perhaps we could identify the strongest pre- dictors of a certain health behaviour and measure them with proxies.

What is more challenging would be to translate Roemer's idea to health states caused by multiple determinants, including health behav- iours. As Roemer himself admits, his proposal is only defined 'if there is a unidimensional kind of "effort" a person can take to lower the proba- bility of suffering the disadvantage in question' (Roemer et al. 1995). A strong correlation between smoking and lung cancer is known, and this strong correlation is the key in Roemer's proposal. Most health behav- iours do not present such a strong correlation with health outcomes, and health is determined by multiple determinants.

In this section, we examined considerations we must make if we derive our judgment on health equity from health determinants. The next three perspectives on health equity focus on different groups of health determinants with complex interactions.

BY SOCIO-ECONOMIC STATUS (SES)

The empirical analysis of health inequity has most often been approached through examination of differences in average health between socio-economic groups. Inequalities in health caused by SES, that is, Group I determinants in table 2.1 above, to many present an intuitive moral concern, and the prevailing view is that health inequali- ties caused by SES are health inequities. Braveman, for example, pro- poses to view that 'pursuing health equity means pursuing the elimina- tion of such health disparities/inequalities' (2006, 180) as 'systematic, potentially avoidable differences in health – or in the major socially determined influences on health – between groups of people who have different relative positions in social hierarchies according to wealth, power, or prestige' (2006, 181).

The classification of health determinants in table 2.1 might help explain a little more about this intuitive concern for health inequalities caused by SES. We might say that society cannot be responsible for things that are nobody's fault. While we might feel sorry, society does not need to assume responsibility for somebody randomly hit by lightning or the old who become frail due to the aging process. In addition, we might think that society should pass no judgments on autonomous decisions its rational citizens make. As we discussed in the previous section, health determinants in the three groups in table 2.1 interact with each other, and all interactions with Group I, social arrangement determinants, would be judged to cause health inequity from this perspective.

Recently philosophers have become interested in health inequalities caused by SES from the perspective of justice.[8] Some try to explain what is wrong about health inequalities caused by SES a little more rigorously by incorporating health into philosophical theories. Here I introduce two such attempts. One is the effort to expand Rawls's theory of justice (1971) as fairness to health, and the other adopting the view of inequity as dominance proposed in Michael Walzer's 'complex equality' (1983).

Above we discussed that we might support a view of strict equality of health outcome if we thought of health as a good resembling political liberty. Health, under the assumption that it is included in the list of social primary goods, might instead be better perceived as a good governed by the difference principle along with income and other goods. Health, like income, is useful for any life plan, and a rational person would want as much of it as possible. The importance of health, unlike political liberty, is not sufficient to justify strict equality. Perceiving health as a difference principle good, we appreciate the importance of health as much as other social primary goods. The governing principle, the difference principle, instructs us that inequality is permissible only if redistribution improves the worst-off's position. Consequently, if health was successfully included in the Rawlsian framework as a difference principle good, we would be concerned only about the average health of the worst-off in health distribution.

The inclusion of health in the list of social primary goods is believed to cause complications and difficulties in Rawls's theory of justice.

Rawls, for example, originally suggests income as the index of the holding of the entire social primary goods, and with that income index we can identify a representative person at the bottom of the basic social structure. If health were included, how should we construct the index of primary goods? Should income alone still be the index? Should health instead be the index? Or should both income and health be a weighted index? Answers to these questions determine who the worst-off are, the poor or the sick.[9] If the latter, contrary to initial expectations, the Rawlsian framework would not help us examine what is wrong about health inequalities caused by SES, which is generally conceptualized and measured by a non-health factor. The difference principle applied to health might intuitively be taken as considering the health of the poor, but there are many issues that need to be resolved before reaching that conclusion.

An alternative philosophical perspective on what is really wrong about health inequalities caused by SES can be sought in Walzer's complex equality (1983). As we touched on very briefly at the end of the introduction, Walzer invites us to think that there are a number of independent spheres of justice, each of them governed by different rules according to the characteristics of the sphere in question and the society of interest. It is possible to develop Walzer's view with regard to health as one sphere and seek its distributional rules. Alternatively, Walzer's view can be developed in a quite different way, based on his view that dominance is unjust. As long as equal political participation and liberty are guaranteed, he argues, inequality in each valued sphere of life does not itself raise a moral concern. What concerns us morally, in his view, is the concentration of burdens and prestige; the rich hold higher social status and are happy and healthy, while the poor endure lower social status and are unhappy and sick. When spheres of life we value correlate with each other, it is difficult to show equal moral respect for all persons. This dominance, Walzer says, should be the heart of our concern for inequality, not inequality in each sphere.

Hausman (n.d. a) introduces this view of Walzer's complex equality to health. Imagine a society where different qualities do not correlate with each other at all – people with disabilities are successful, for example, politically, professionally, and economically. Health would not be equally distributed in such a society, but is it a problem? It may not be, if our fundamental concern is equal moral respect for each person. What bothers us is that the healthy are more likely to be successful and the sick less likely to be successful in other valued spheres of life.

Although there may be some intrinsic value in health equality, Hausman suggests that, should we be concerned with moral status, we would be especially concerned about the existence and magnitude of correlations between health status and SES.

Strictly speaking, this view of inequity as dominance is concerned with the correlation between health and SES but not the causal relationship between them. Suppose that the only health difference we observe between the poor and the rich is due to a mysterious genetic disease concentrated among the poor. We do not know why it is concentrated among the poor and have found no evidence that any condition of the poor invites this genetic disease. Its concentration among the poor is simply a misfortune. The inequity-as-dominance view would still be concerned about this correlation between poor health and low SES, while the Rawlsian perspective or any other views that care only about health inequalities caused by the basic social structure would not. In the actual mechanism of dominance, however, distributions of goods are unlikely to correlate with each other just by chance. It is thus reasonable, even for the view of inequity as dominance, to consider that health inequalities caused by SES are inequitable.

BY FACTORS BEYOND INDIVIDUAL CONTROL

Although health inequity is most often (intuitively) defined as health inequalities caused by SES, some researchers pay attention to other determinants. Here we look at a view acknowledging the value of choice in producing health. Le Grand, for example, defines health equity as follows: 'If an individual's ill-health results from factors beyond his or her control, then the situation is inequitable; if it results from factors within his or her control, then it is equitable' (1991, 114). Similarly, Whitehead writes: 'Judgments on which situations are unfair will vary from place to place and from time to time, but one widely used criterion is the degree of *choice* involved. Where people have little or no choice of living and working conditions, the resulting health differences are more likely to be considered unjust than those resulting from health risks that were chosen voluntarily' (1992, 433, original emphasis). The idea echoed in both the views of Le Grand and Whitehead is the appreciation of freedom or autonomous decision making. Health is important and special but not so special as to justify a constraint on the freedom to obtain or exercise it. The price of the freedom is individual responsibility.

Central to this perspective of health inequity as health inequality caused by factors beyond individual control is the determination of factors beyond individual control. Recall our classification of health determinants in table 2.1. If one could categorize determinants into three mutually exclusive groups, then Group I health inequalities (social responsibility) and Group III inequalities (nobody's fault) would be considered to be inequitable. It might appear absurd that such health inequalities as men's generally shorter lifespan than women's, or the elderly's generally more frail health than the young's, are regarded as inequitable. One might wish to reconsider how biological variations should be incorporated in this perspective.

However biological variations are considered, as we discussed above, both conceptually and empirically, it is very difficult to identify factors beyond individual control. Note that the quick solution of looking at the average health in each socio-economic group is not appropriate for this perspective. The averaging strategy misses such a health determinant as a random genetic disease whose incidence does not relate to SES. This perspective on health equity would regard such a random genetic disease as a cause of health equity, because a random genetic disease is still a factor beyond individual control despite having no relation to SES. Yet its occurrence would not be picked up by looking only at the average health in each group.[10] If the averaging strategy is not appropriate for this equity perspective, we may have to instead adopt something like Roemer's proposal, whose difficulties we have already discussed. The choice argument might sound attractive at first sight, but many issues need to be resolved before it can be implemented.

BY FACTORS AMENABLE TO HUMAN INTERVENTIONS

In measuring health inequality for *The World Health Report 2000*, Gakidou, Murray, and Frenk (1999) proposed another perspective, which denies that only health inequalities caused by social factors qualify as inequitable. Specifically, they paid attention to genetic factors. They consider that health inequalities caused by genetics are also inequitable. Their primary concern is not whether health inequalities are caused by social factors, but rather, whether the causes are susceptible to human intervention. In their perspective on health equity, health inequalities caused by factors amenable to human interventions are inequitable (Asada and Hedemann 2002).

Which of the three group determinants in table 2.1 is amenable to human intervention? Health inequalities caused by the Group I determinants, the basic social structure, are by definition amenable to human intervention, so they are inequitable in the perspective of Gakidou, Murray, and Frenk. They take the position that true personal choice in health production scarcely exists and argue that health inequalities caused by informed choice 'should not be excluded' from the equity consideration (Gakidou, Murray, and Frenk 2000, 46). Thus, they would judge health inequalities caused by the Group II determinants (choice) as inequitable. Judgment on the Group III determinants (nobody's fault) is a little more complex. From the perspective of Gakidou, Murray, and Frenk, what is important in judging these determinants is not whether the determinant of health inequality of interest falls into this category but whether any resulting health inequality was mitigated when we had the means. For example, health inequality caused by a genetic disease whose incidence is random but whose treatment is established would be considered as inequitable. Similarly, if we found a way to prolong men's lifespan as long as women's, then health inequality due to the lack of this action may be regarded as inequitable.[11]

HOW DIFFERENT ARE THESE THREE PERSPECTIVES?

So far, we have looked at three different perspectives on health equity, each of which focuses on particular causes of health inequalities and considers them to be inequitable. In this subsection I highlight differences between these three perspectives with examples. Despite the unsolved issues of health in the Rawlsian framework, here I follow the general intuitive interpretation of the view of inequity as inequalities caused by SES: health inequalities caused by social causes are inequitable. Consider the following health inequalities:

- Health inequality 1: Socio-economic gradient in health.
- Health inequality 2: Health inequality caused by skydiving based on free, informed choice.
- Health inequality 3: Health inequality caused by genetic disease randomly occurring (with no relation to SES). An intervention exists that completely cures it.
- Health inequality 4: Health inequality caused by sex (for example, men tend to die younger than women).
- Health inequality 5: Health inequality caused by gender (that is, socially shaped characteristics based on biological sex). For example, men's health is more likely to deteriorate than women's due to violence.

Table 2.2
Examples of health determinants and equity perspectives

Health inequality caused by	Health determinant classification	Perspective		
		SES	Individual control	Amenable to human interventions
1 SES	Responsibility of society (Group I)	✔	✔	✔
2 Sky diving	Choice (Group II)			✔
3 Random genetic disease	Nobody's fault (Group III)		✔	✔
4 Sex	Nobody's fault (Group III)		✔	
5 Gender	Responsibility of society (Group I) x nobody's fault (Group III)	✔	✔	✔

✔: regards as inequitable
blank: does not regard as inequitable

Which health inequalities do the three perspectives regard as inequitable? Table 2.2 summarizes their responses. The perspective that defines health inequalities caused by SES as inequitable would not consider health inequalities caused by random genetic disease or sex to be inequitable. In this view, society cannot be responsible for random misfortune and distribution of such a natural good as sex. The perspective that defines health inequality caused by factors beyond individual control as inequitable, on the other hand, regards health inequalities caused by all factors apart from skydiving as they are beyond individual control.[12] The view of health inequity as health inequality caused by factors amenable to human interventions proposed by Gakidou, Murray, and Frenk is as expansive as the perspective focusing on individual control: it judges that only health inequality caused by sex is outside of the equity consideration. The perspective proposed by Gakidou, Murray, and Frenk was criticized for diverting attention from health inequality caused by SES.[13] Because health inequality caused by SES is amenable to human interventions, this claim is, at least at the conceptual level, false.

Focusing on Level

To investigate which health distributions are inequitable, many health sciences researchers seem to believe that we must examine health determinants. Another approach is possible, however: we instead focus on the level of health.

In her thought-provoking paper 'What is the Point of Equality?' Elizabeth Anderson warns that recent egalitarian thinking focuses too much on 'compensating people for underserved bad luck' (1999, 288). Examining how people obtained a certain quantity of essential resources in life or how they reached a certain level of well-being, in her view, does not show respect to persons. She remarks that 'what citizens ultimately owe one another is the social conditions of freedoms people need to function as equal citizens' (1999, 320). These social conditions may be broken down into a variety of spheres, including health. Society in this case might be concerned about whether each person satisfies the minimally adequate level of health regardless of how each person realizes her health. People are not allowed to make trade-offs between health and other goods below the minimally adequate level of health, because this minimally adequate level is considered to be invaluable as a multi-purpose good that is useful for any life plans. Above this minimally adequate level, however, depending on one's preferences and conceptions of a good life, people can trade off health with other goods. This, in other words, means that health inequalities above this minimally adequate level of health are not of moral concern, and, thus, do not need to be measured.

We can trace this idea of the minimally adequate level of health in two philosophical theories: Norman Daniels's normal species functioning (1985) and Martha Nussbaum's version of the capability approach (2000).[14] They are introduced respectively below.

NORMAL SPECIES FUNCTIONING

To identify the health care needs (Daniels 1985) and, later, health needs (Daniels, Kennedy, and Kawachi 2004) for which a society ought to provide assistance, Daniels introduces the idea called species-typical normal functioning. Acknowledging the difficulty involved in conceptualizing health, Daniels opts for a narrow, 'biomedical' model of health as the best strategy to define health needs. The basic idea of this biomedical model is that 'health is the absence of disease, and diseases ... are *deviations from the natural functional organization of a typical member of a species'* (1985, 28, original emphasis). Maintaining species-typical normal functioning is important, because 'impairments of normal species functioning reduce the range of opportunity open to the individual in which he may construct his "plan of life" or "conception of the good"' (1985, 27). Opportunity, in his idea, is much more general and expansive than in Rawls's view, in which the opportunity is only the one related to office and job. Like Rawls, however, Daniels admits that people with different talents and skills possess different opportunities. Society ought to guarantee species-typical normal functioning to each of its citizens so they can enjoy full potential according to their talents and skills.

Daniels emphasizes that the normal opportunity range is socially relative. The range of opportunity a society provides to its citizens differs according to its historical and technological development, wealth, and culture (1985, 33). How, then, might species-typical normal functioning, which appears to be universal to all human species given its derivation from the biological construct of humans, respond to the social relativity of the normal opportunity range? One way to answer this question is to understand species-typical normal functioning as a list of different types of normal species functioning, which is the same for every individual irrespective of her society, but the weight for each functioning, that is, the relative importance of each functioning, may be different in different societies. Take the example of reproduction. Reproduction is likely to be included in the list of normal species functionings. Suppose that we were interested in how many people lack this particular normal species functioning in India and the United States. Given how important reproduction is to enhance one's opportunity range in each society, we might want to give different weights to reproduction in these countries.[15]

CAPABILITY APPROACH (NUSSBAUM)

Two scholars independently developed a so-called capability approach, albeit following a period of collaboration. As is well known, Amartya Sen fashioned the idea of capability in development economics (1992; 1993), and, though perhaps less known, Martha Nussbaum in philosophy (2000). When working together in 1980s, they recognized a 'striking resemblance' in each other's idea (Nussbaum 2000, 11). Their ideas, however, were not identical and did not merge after that collaborative period. I believe it is Nussbaum's version of the capability approach that has greater promise in health equity research and has already been introduced in the health context (for example, Stronks and Gunning-Schepers 1993), although it is frequently referred to as Sen's capability approach (Pereira 1993; Peter 2001). Before getting into this detail, let me start by explaining the essentials of the capability approach shared both by Sen and Nussbaum.

The capability approach may be best viewed as a position somewhere between the welfarist and resourcist. Trying to equalize welfare or well-being is too much, because society should not be responsible for what people freely choose to do in their lives. Trying to equalize resources, on the other hand, is too little, as it does not take sufficient care of the diversity in our internal characteristics. Pregnant women, for example, have different nutritional needs from others, and newly arrived immigrants would not benefit from public services without a proper translator of language and culture. For various reasons, people are different in the power to convert resources given to exploit the freedom they enjoy. Focusing only on providing resources is not enough. The capability approach instead pays attention to the relationship between a person and resources (Sen 1992, 27).

The capability approach expresses this idea in its own terminologies. Functionings are things we do, for example, reading and writing. Capabilities are abilities that enable such functionings, for example, literacy. The proper focus of egalitarians is not that people actually do and are (functionings) but what they can do (capabilities). This view is thus commonly referred to as the capability approach. Note that functioning in the capability approach and in Daniels's species-typical normal functioning idea are not the same. I will discuss the difference in detail in chapter 3.

Sen is deliberately ambiguous about what capabilities consist in and limits himself to saying that each individual should have an 'equivalent' capability set. Moreover, even though some scholars believe that health might be better perceived as a capability or subset of capabilities (Pereira 1993; Peter 2001), Sen himself often uses health as an example of functioning (for example, Sen 1992, 39). Even if Sen agreed that health was a capability, it would still be unclear whether he would also agree to separate health from a capability set and independently examine its distribution.

Nussbaum's approach differs from Sen's. She provides a list of 'central human functional capabilities,' which includes the length of life (Life), physical health-adjusted quality of life (Bodily Health), and mental health-adjusted quality of life (spread into different categories, depending on how one defines mental health: Senses, Imagination, and Thought; Emotions; and Practical Reason) (2000, 78–80). In short, health, in the most general sense we are so far using the term in this project, is recognized as one of the central human functional capabilities in her view. And Nussbaum's version of the capability approach implies the basic minimum that society ought to ensure for its citizens. A word of caution is in order regarding the interpretation of this basic minimum. Nussbaum favours its recognition with 'reference to an idea of human worth or dignity,' instead of the literal interpretation that below it people are better off if dead (2000, 73). This is compatible with the view of Anderson, who proposes what she calls democratic equality as an expansion of the core idea of the capability approach. She writes that 'democratic equality guarantees not effective access to equal levels of functioning but effective access to levels of functioning sufficient to stand as an equal in society' (Anderson 1999, 318).

CONCLUDING NOTE ON THE VIEW OF THE MINIMALLY ADEQUATE LEVEL OF HEALTH

There are at least three major challenges to the idea of the minimally adequate level of health. First, how do we define the minimum level of health? When the just distribution of health care was passionately discussed some decades ago, many scholars (for example, Buchanan 1984; Harris 1999; Veatch 1991) and activists tried to define the minimally adequate level of health care but in vain. Might defining the minimally adequate level of health be so destined?[16] I do not know the answer, but the theories seem to be attractive enough that I think it is worth trying. Popular perspectives on health equity based on causal paths are not flawless either; it seems fair simply to say that no account of health equity is without difficulty.

Indeed, most of the equity accounts introduced as a reasonable relaxation of strict equality of health outcome, both by cause and level, still suffer from the problem of cost. If one were serious about these views and tried to equalize health accordingly, society would go bankrupt. The equity goals are not feasible. One might argue that this is actually not a question of health equity.[17] In this project, we focus on health equity. But in the real world of health policy-making, we would not be concerned only about health equity. There would be additional goals of population health just as important as equity, most notably, efficiency. How much closer should we get to an infeasible health equity goal? The answer needs to be sought by balancing our value of equity with that of other ideals.

Among the five equity perspectives one way or another modified from the view of strict equality of health outcome, the one that does not bankrupt society is the view of equity as equality in health caused by SES. The reason why this perspective does not raise the problem of cost to the same extent is not intrinsic to the nature of the theory but relates to the question of among whom health equity should be sought. I postpone this discussion until the section of the unit of analysis in chapter 3.

Finally, perhaps the most crucial challenge for the view of equity as satisfying the minimally adequate level of health is the problem of the 'hopelessly sick.' However we define the minimum basic level of health, there will always be someone who cannot satisfy the minimum even with the cutting-edge medical technology and knowledge. Note that we are not merely talking here about the cost of helping those below the minimum level; even with unlimited resources on earth, there would be conditions that we would not be able to help.[18] How would the view of the minimally adequate level of health respond to such situations? This is a critical question for this perspective to survive as an attractive account of health equity.

2.3 Health Inequality as an Indicator of Social Justice

Recall our discussion in the introduction that one might be interested in health inequity because health can be considered to be an indicator of general social justice. Directly corresponding to this view, some researchers define and measure health inequity accordingly. Unlike in the first category of equity as equality in health, this perspective is not concerned about which health – by causal path or level – we should focus on as the equalization target. Its primary interest is not so much in our value of health in itself. It instead pays more attention to the health distribution as a whole as carrying important information about general social justice.

Sen, for example, proposes to use mortality as a supplement to the conventional economic indicators for its '(1) intrinsic importance (since a longer life is valued in itself), (2) enabling significance (since being alive is a necessary condition for our capabilities), and (3) associative relevance (since many other valuable achievements relate – negatively – to mortality rates)' (1998, 22). More specifically on (3), Sen argues that such policy issues as epidemiological environment, access to health care and health insurance, basic education, and social inequalities are all

reflected in mortality information (1998, 23). The reasons why he rec-
ommends mortality rather than morbidity or other health indicators are
data availability and methodological challenges that measurement of
health faces. As the field of health outcome measurement develops, his
proposal can be generalizable to other health indicators.

A similar view can be traced in a proposal by Daniels, Kennedy, and
Kawachi (2000). They are intrigued by an interesting coincidence that
the social primary goods that Rawls suggests in his theory of justice as
fairness happen to be important determinants of health. 'Social justice
is good for our health' they therefore claim (Daniels, Kennedy, and
Kawachi 2000, 33). In this view, the primary concern is just distribution
of social primary goods. But it is possible to view the coincidence
between the social primary goods and health determinants in another
way: we may be able to use the distribution of health as an indicator of
a just society.[19]

2.4 Three Egalitarian Reasons Revisited

Let us recall the three reasons introduced in the introduction why one
might be morally interested in health distribution:

1 Health is a special good, so we are morally concerned about its
   distribution.
2 We are interested in the general pursuit of justice, and health is
   included in it. There are a number of important goods that we care
   about in the general pursuit of justice.
   2a There is a good reason to focus on health among other
      important goods.
   2b There is no good reason to focus on health among other
      important goods.
3 Health can be used as an indicator of general social justice.

From the measurement perspective, (1) and (2a) are indistinguishable;
if we took either of these perspectives, we would only measure health. If
we took (2b), on the other hand, we would always want to measure
health distribution along with distributions of other goods. These
reasons are the basis of different perspectives on health equity we
looked at in this chapter. What exactly is the connection? Figure 2.1
summarizes this point.

Let me start from the bottom. If one were morally concerned about

Figure 2.1 Summary of chapter 2

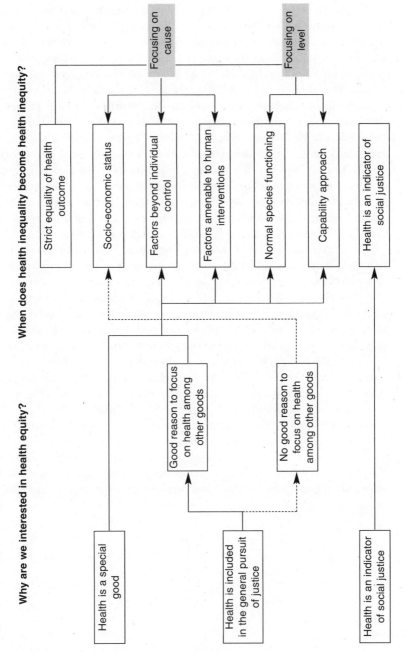

health distribution in the belief that health could be used as an indicator of general social justice, one would consequently say that health inequality as a whole was inequity in the sense that it reflected social injustice. Suppose next that one was interested in pursuing justice in general, believed that health should be included in that general pursuit of justice, but considered that health is only as special as other important goods. In this case, one would say that health inequality caused by the basic social structure is inequitable. If, on the other hand, one believed that health was special to some degree, one would be interested in health distribution irrespective of its relationships to other goods. One might say that health inequalities caused by such certain determinants as factors beyond individual control or factors amenable to human interventions are inequities. Or, alternatively, one might instead be interested in whether everyone in a population reaches a certain level of health irrespective of how it was realized.

These are connections between egalitarian reasons to be interested in health distribution and its different perspectives of health equity. In the introduction, we also looked at another ethical reason to be concerned about health distribution, that is, the utilitarian perspective. It is, for example, often said that we should be concerned about health inequality because it has a negative effect on improving the overall health of the population. From the utilitarian perspective, which health distribution is inequitable? Strictly speaking, it should be the one that has the strongest negative impact on the overall health of the population. The utilitarian perspective is sometimes used as a reason why we might want to reduce health inequality caused by SES (Charlton 1994; Woodward and Kawachi 2000, 2001), but there has been no evidence that this is the type of health inequality that has the strongest effect on the overall level of population health. In this regard, this chapter, which shows that there are many different ways to focus on particular health inequalities, might also be useful for those who support the utilitarian perspective.

3 What Measurement Choices Must Be Faced to Measure Health Inequity?

3.1 Introduction

The previous two chapters familiarized us with different perspectives on health equity. Some of us might be attracted to a certain perspective or might develop an account of health equity of our own based on discussion in these two chapters. Now imagine that we wish to think of measuring health equity according to a chosen perspective. To operationalize an equity perspective as a measurement strategy, whichever it may be, there are further issues to be considered. We have, for example, been talking about health only vaguely, but what exactly is the health we are talking about?

In this chapter, we discuss some of the issues bridging a theory and measurement strategy. We look at issues about health (for example, the question of which aspects of health we should consider), the unit of time, and the unit of analysis. Some might think that these are purely measurement questions based on data availability, but I argue that when our interest in health inequality is moral, moral considerations should also influence measurement strategy. The unit of time, for example, may be a data availability issue, but at the same time, it better reflects our view of the time period within which we are concerned about health equity. Similarly, the unit of analysis raises the question of among whom health should equally be distributed as well as what kind of data we have the access to.

3.2 Issues about Health

We cannot measure health inequity without measuring health. Health is a multi-dimensional concept, without an as yet generally agreed definition. The field of measurement of health is a fascinating, rapidly devel-

oping research area, and measurement of health inequity must go hand
in hand with the development of health measurement. The focus of this
book, nonetheless, is not measurement of health but that of health
inequity. Below I discuss some of the issues concerning health measurement that are of particular interest for our purpose.

Health as Functionality

Health is notoriously difficult to define. A wide range of definitions of
health can be understood on a continuum axis (Evans and Stoddart
1990). At one end is the narrowest understanding of health: the
absence of disease, pain, disability, or death. At the other end is the
broadest, all-encompassing view defined by the WHO: 'a state of
complete physical, mental, and social well-being, and not merely the
absence of disease or injury' (1946). We all agree that the definition of
health is located somewhere between these two extremes but have yet
to agree where exactly that is.

Reviewing different perspectives on health equity in the previous two
chapters, we did not specify what health exactly is. Perhaps it is too big
a task for this book to define health in general, so instead we might ask:
what aspect of health should we consider when we think of health
equity? To examine this question, let us recall reasons why we are
morally concerned about health distribution. We discussed in the introduction that health is special in at least two ways. First, health in itself is
one component of welfare or well-being. Second, health is a multi-
purpose good that is useful for any life plan. We may not agree on how
special health is. These characteristics of health nevertheless form the
fundamental basis of our moral interest in health distribution. When we
pay attention to health in this way, the name of a disease does not have
much importance. What is relevant to our interest is what a person can
or cannot do. It may also matter whether a person exhibits general
symptoms such as pain or anxiety. A different disease category per se
does not affect the level of health-related welfare or the potential use of
health as a multi-purpose resource. Instead, functionality, disability, or
general symptoms determine the health-related welfare level and the
use of health as a multi-purpose resource.

The focus on functionality is compatible with the general trend in
the health measurement field. As functional measures, health science
researchers would immediately list the ADL (Activities of Daily Living),
which assesses independence in such basic daily living abilities as

bathing, dressing, and eating, and the IADL (Instrumental Activities of Daily Living), which assesses such applied aspects of daily living as difficulties in shopping, cooking, and managing money (McDowell and Newll 1996, 48–50). In addition, many of the cutting-edge general health status measures also look at functionality as well as general symptoms, although they may not be perceived as functional measures.[1] A person with perfect health in the EQ-5D, one of the leading measures of health status especially popular in Europe, for example, has no problems with mobility, self-care, the performance of usual activities, pain or discomfort, and anxiety or depression (McDowell and Newll 1996, 481).

Functioning, functionality, or function covers a wide range of concepts, and it is sometimes confusing what it really means. The capability approach (see section 2.2 in chapter 2), for example, uses the term 'functioning' for actual doing and being, as opposed to capabilities, which suggest a potential to do an activity or to be in a condition. Daniels's functioning (see section 2.2 in chapter 2), on the other hand, appears to be more biological in his usage of species-typical normal functioning. How exactly do these functionings differ? In addition, how do they relate to the functionality of the conventional usage in the health measurement field?

To classify the wide-ranging concept of functionality, the International Classification of Functioning, Disability and Health (ICF) proposed by the WHO is useful (2001). The ICF divides functionality in two components: (1) body functions and structures, and (2) activities and participation. It defines these as follows:

- Body functions are the physiological functions of body systems (including psychological functions).
- Body structures are anatomical parts of the body such as organs, limbs, and their components.
- Activity is the execution of a task or action by an individual.
- Participation is involvement in a life situation.

In addition, activities and participation are characterized in either of two ways: capacity or performance, defined as follows:

- Capacity is an individual's ability to execute a task or action in a 'standardized' environment, in other words, the environmentally adjusted ability of the individual.

Figure 3.1   Concepts of functionality

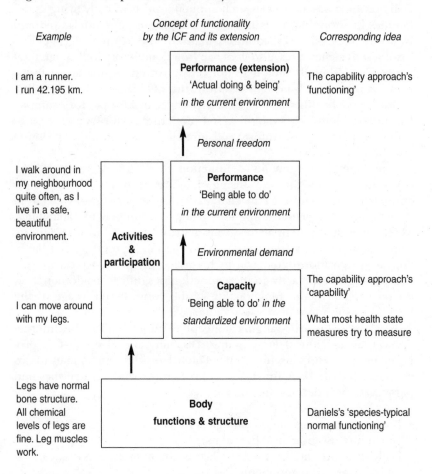

- Performance is what an individual does in his or her current environment.

The difference between capacity and performance, according to the ICF classification, is a demand imposed by the living environment. Suppose that two people are assessed as being able to walk around in a 'standardized' environment. Various environmental factors positively or negatively affect their capacity level and, consequently, produce different levels of performance. One of them, for example, may not be able to walk around much because her neighbourhood is dangerous. The other may need to walk a great distance every day because the closest well is miles away.

Note that the ICF does not classify personal factors, such as motivation, which could also create a difference between capacity and performance. It is not only environmental demands but also personal freedom that determine what an individual actually does in her environment. People who exhibit a capacity for walking make different decisions on how to use that capacity. Some might devote themselves to sedentary academic work, while others might wish to become marathon runners.

Adopting the ICF and its extension regarding personal factors, figure 3.1 summarizes various concepts of functionality we have discussed. The focus of the first level of functionality is the human body, and functionality at this level concerns the body functions and structure as a member of the human species. Daniels's 'species-typical normal functioning' is the functionality at this level. The second level of functionality is the concept of capacity in the ICF, and this corresponds to 'capability' in the context of the capability approach.[2] 'Functioning' in the capability approach matches the extended concept of performance, as the capability approach accepts individuals' freedom to decide what to do and how to be.

The direct correspondence between this understanding of functionality and the capability approach is unfortunate. It might give the wrong impression that this understanding of functionality can only be reasonably applied to the perspective on health equity influenced by the capability approach. But it is the acknowledgment of health as a multipurpose resource that enables us reasonably to focus on health as functionality.

Now let us think of these different levels of functionality for a marathon runner. Running 42.195 km is her extended performance, which is the execution of a task that she chooses to do in her living environment. Her mobility is a capacity assessed in the standardized environment, which enables her to walk around her neighbourhood if her surrounding environment allows (performance in the ICF context) and to run a marathon if she wants to (extended performance). This capacity is supported by the most fundamental functioning, body functions and structure. In order for her legs to be able to move her around, for example, they must have the normal bone structure and effective chemical interactions that assist general muscle movements.

Neither health status measures (for example, EQ-5D and Health Utilities Index or HUI) nor functional measures (for example, ADL and IADL) ask people about specific performances in their particular environments, for example, whether they run a marathon. Rather, these health measures focus on activities and performance, for example, being able to move around, hear, or see. Although it is often not obvious whether cutting-edge health status measures intend to assess capacity or performance, it is perhaps capacity rather than performance that they intend to assess. Chatterji et al., for example, recently developed a health status measure for the World Health Survey incorporating the ICF classification and advocate capacity: 'we would not say that an individual with a hearing impairment is healthier simply because she avoids noisy gatherings' (2002, 11). Capacities are prerequisites for whatever specific task one might end up doing due to environmental pressure or the free exercise of one's own will. From the perspective on health equity, this focus on capacity seems to be the right one. The concept of capacity appears to capture our value of health as a multipurpose resource useful for any life plans.[3]

Many of the currently available health status measures suffer from the ceiling effect: the majority of people assessed classify themselves in the highest category of the health level. It seems that we know how to separate the sick but not the healthy. Using such health status measures for health inequity analysis, we would not observe much inequity. Is this a problem? David Feeny and his colleagues, for example, discuss the possibility of seeking 'supra-normal health,' that is, further to categorize the healthy, which is usually capped as 'full' or 'perfect' health in currently available health status measures (Feeny et al. 1995, 497). But they themselves acknowledge that the ceiling effect is unavoidable when we intend to measure capacity instead of performance. If what we wish to know is a capacity level that opens up performance options to us and enables us to carry out a chosen performance, we may not need to know more than the 'full' or 'perfect' health assessed by the health status measures. What we should want to measure is not whether inequality is ubiquitous but whether meaningful inequity exists, regardless of the degree of health inequity.[4]

To conclude this section, let us see what consequences the different focus of functionality might bring in health inequity measurement. In chapter 2, I introduced two types of equity perspective on the minimally adequate level of health. One uses Daniels's species-typical normal functioning view, and the other the capability approach. Now it is clear that these two perspectives actually focus on different types of functionality. Normal species functioning is concerned about functionality as a body function and structure, while the capability approach looks at functionality as capacity. What consequences does this difference bring? Let us take the famous example of short stature (Allen and Fost 1990, 18).

- Johnny is a short eleven-year-old boy with documented growth hormone deficiency resulting from a brain tumour. His parents are of average height. His predicted adult height without growth hormone treatment is approximately 160 cm (5 feet 3 inches).
- Billy is a short eleven-year-old boy with normal growth hormone secretion according to current testing methods. However, his parents are extremely short, and he has a predicted adult height of 160 cm (5 feet 3 inches).

How does each of these two perspectives regard the short stature of Johnny and Billy? In the normal species functioning view, short stature would be of concern if it resulted from 'deviations from the natural functional organization of a typical member of a species' (Daniels 1985, 28). Johnny is short because his growth hormone secretion is not 'normal' for a typical member of his species. But Billy's short stature cannot be demonstrably linked to such a biological abnormality. Consequently, the normal species functioning view would judge, in terms of stature, that Johnny does not satisfy the minimally adequate level of health but Billy does. The capability approach, on the other hand, would be concerned about the lack of capacity resulting from a short stature. In this case, there would be no distinction between Johnny and Billy.[5]

Health Determinants, Expectation, and Outcome

Any aspect of health, including functionality, has a complex production process. Unless we understand it and distinguish health determinants, expectation, and outcome, any discussion of health equity will remain vague.

Let us start by understanding someone's health production process as follows: a person has certain internal and external resources (for

Figure 3.2   The Evans-Stoddart model of determinants of health

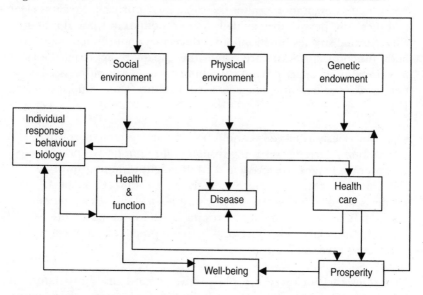

Source: Evans and Stoddart (1990), p. 1359, fig. 5, reprinted with permission from Elsevier.

example, biological bodily function and physical environment, respectively) that together predict her health expectation. With choice (for example, exercise) and chance (for example, being hit by lightning), she realizes her health outcome.

Various factors play roles in health production. Robert Evans and Gregory Stoddart propose a highly influential model of determinants of health as reproduced in figure 3.2 (1990, 1359). Their model represents the ideas that health is more than the mere state of the absence of disease and injury and that determinants of health are more than health care. The model consists of nine categories: disease, health care, health and function, social environment, physical environment, genetic endowment, individual response (behaviour and biology), well-being, and prosperity. Each of these nine categories has a rich internal structure and relates in a complex way to the others. Given its conceptual complexity and the empirical challenges it provides, Stoddard calls this model a 'fantasy equation' (1995).

Figure 3.3 illustrates how health determinants in the Evans-Stoddart

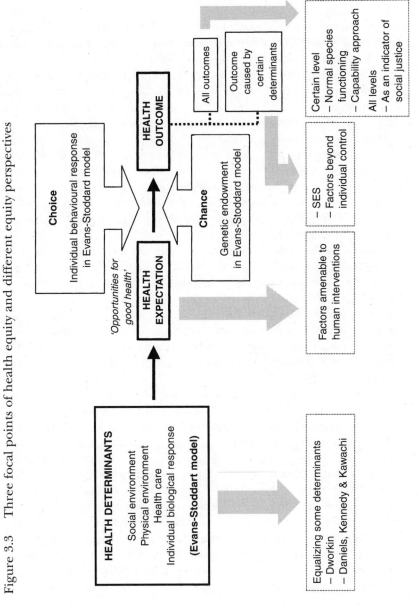

Figure 3.3   Three focal points of health equity and different equity perspectives

model affect health expectation and outcome. Here, 'resources' in the philosophical equality literature are reshaped as health determinants. Note that in the Evans-Stoddart model, anything that determines health – both health expectation and outcome – are called 'determinants of health.' Some determinants of health (social and physical environment, individual biological responses, and health care) together predict health expectation. Other determinants (individual behavioural response and chance, which is not included in the Evans-Stoddart model[6]) alter health expectation as to outcome. Furthermore, 'socio-economic status' is an umbrella category consisting of some determinants or portions of some determinants that are socially arranged.

When we talk about health equity, it is important to be clear about which focal point of health – health determinants, expectation, or outcome – we are thinking of. To put it differently, it is a good exercise to examine which of the three might be the best focal point of a certain perspective on health equity and why. Figure 3.3 also summarizes which focal point of health is chosen by the different perspectives on health equity from chapter 2.[7]

Most of the perspectives on health equity we looked at in chapter 2 select health outcome as the focal point. As we saw at the beginning of chapter 2, aiming for the strict equality of health outcome is problematic, and most perspectives on health equity look at certain parts of health outcome one way or another. The perspective of health inequality as an indicator of social justice does focus on all levels of health outcome caused by all possible determinants, but as we discussed in chapter 2, this perspective does not look at this entire health outcome as the good to be equalized.

Health expectation is sometimes referred to as 'opportunities for good health' and considered to be an attractive focal point of health in the health equity discussion (Chang 2002; Gakidou, Murray, and Frenk 2000; Veatch 1991). As we discussed in our examination of health determinants in chapter 2, it is often thought that chance determinants should be dropped in the equity discussion as they are nobody's responsibility, and choice determinants should similarly be excluded because we appreciate the autonomous decision of a rational citizen. And some researchers, for example, Gakidou, Murray, and Frenk (2000), argue that when we wish only to focus on a health outcome produced by factors other than chance and choice determinants, our health focus is technically the same as our health expectation. As the phrase 'opportunity for good health' expresses, if this were true, health expectation would be a handy concept for the aspect of health we wish to distribute equally among people.

The perspective on health equity proposed by Gakidou, Murray, and Frenk (2000) for the WHO health inequality index is thus an example of opting for health expectation as the focal point. It defines health expectation as the expected survival years with full health, and its view that we should aim for equalizing health expectation is supported by the following three arguments. First, Gakidou, Murray, and Frenk believe that health inequalities caused by factors amenable to human interventions are of moral concern. Second, they do not think that personal choice really exists in health production. Lastly, they are not interested in health inequalities caused by random chance events. Putting these three arguments together, they focus on health expectation. The focus on health expectation unfortunately presents both conceptual and methodological problems.

In order to know the health expectation of somebody, we need all the information that is relevant to health determinants. We need to know, for example, the sex, race or ethnicity, education, income, occupation, physical environment, and nationality of this person. By obtaining the information from people who share these characteristics and have already lived their lives, we can make an assumption of how these characteristics are most likely to influence this person's health. The combination of all of these predictions is the health expectation for this person. Theoretically, it is possible to come up with the health expectation for a person. But in practice the health expectation for an individual is most likely to be some sort of approximation based on the health expectation for a particular group of people (Hausman, Asada, and Hedemann 2002).

This suggests that health expectation can reasonably be defined and measured only for a group of individuals but probably not for an individual. And, thinking further, from where does the information concerning the health expectation for a group of individuals come? It comes from the health outcome of a group of individuals who share the same characteristics of the group whose health expectation is of interest. Is there then any difference between the health expectation for a group sharing a certain characteristic and the health outcome of that group? 'Health expectation' may give a sense of looking forward, and similarly 'health outcome' a sense of looking backward, but how different are they in practical application? This argument is old in demography. What is the point, for example, in looking at life expectancy for a

group instead of the average life years lived of that group? It is of course
useful to focus on expectation rather than outcome, for example,
smoothing over observation-to-observation outliers. But perhaps the
attraction of health expectation may not be all that the expression
'opportunities for good health' implies.

Moreover, the problem of the focus on health expectation in the
WHO health inequity perspective is not only methodological but also
conceptual. For the sake of argument, let us suppose that the health
expectation for an individual can be reasonably measured. By looking
at the health expectation for an individual, then, exactly what type of
chance is excluded? Recall our discussion on genetics as a chance determinant in chapter 2. I pointed out that genetics is not exactly the same
as other chance events, such as being hit by lightning, since the acquisition of the chance happens at the beginning of life. When Gakidou,
Murray, and Frenk remark on the health expectation for an individual,
what kind of individual do they have in mind? Common sense informs
us that each individual possesses 'predetermined' chances, or genetics.
There is always someone in a population who has an incurable genetic
disease. To obtain a gene causing an incurable disease is of course a
matter of chance, but that chance cannot be excluded by looking at the
health expectation for an individual. In other words, one can never
expect that health expectation or 'opportunities for good health' will be
equal.

In chapter 2, we also briefly looked at the view in which we equalize
health determinants rather than expectation or outcome. Usually the
reason why people holding this view[8] are interested in equalizing health
determinants is not that it improves health equity, but because their
interest in health equity is secondary. Their primary interest is in equalizing important goods, which happen also to be important health determinants, and their equal distributions coincidentally improve health
equity. One might find it strange that the focal point of health equity
could be health determinants, but it is actually a difficult question why
the focal point should be health expectation or outcome rather than
determinants.

Medical Technologies, Non-human Aids, Human Assistance, and
Accommodating Environmental Factors

One can assess functionality and general symptoms with or without
medical technologies (for example, medication, laser surgery, or a pacemaker), non-human aids (for example, eyeglasses or a wheelchair),

human assistance (for example, the help of another person), and accommodating environmental factors (for example, a barrier-free physical environment). These distinctions are important in health inequity analysis because they could change the assessment of health and touch on the fundamental question of what health is.

To illustrate the issues I raise in this section, I start with a hypothetical case.

Mai was born to a poor family in rural Cambodia. At the age of five, a landmine blew off one of her arms and paralysed her legs. Because her family were farmers living in a poor rural area, they could not afford an artificial arm for her and could only occasionally borrow an old wheelchair from a community assistance centre. Mai's physical activities totally depended on the help of her family members, who were usually very busy earning a living in any way possible.

At the age of ten, Mai was adopted by a wealthy Japanese couple. Upon moving to Japan, she was provided with an artificial arm and an electric wheelchair, which ensured her mobility, although she still required human assistance for many daily activities, including getting in and out of the wheelchair. Mai's adoptive parents were loving, and Mai, with her cheerful nature and intelligence, flourished in her new home. Her life in Japan was nevertheless still tough. She always needed to fight to study in a 'normal' school for 'normal' children, could seldom use public transportation, and was never sure which restaurants would 'accept' her as a welcome customer.

Frustrated by the social barriers she encountered in Japanese society, at the age of nineteen Mai moved to Berkeley, California, the birthplace of the disability movement in North America. There, her opportunities dramatically expanded. The city provided a personal attendant and accessible public transportation so she could live independently, while the university warmly accepted her as a hard-working student.

Is Mai's health different in Cambodia, Japan, and the United States? Leaving aside obviously important cross-cultural issues, let us assume the legitimacy of using the same health status measure to assess Mai's health in three different countries. Should we assess Mai's health with or without an artificial arm, an electric wheelchair, societal support, and the accommodating physical environment?

A MODEL AND PROBLEM STATEMENT

Mai's case permits us the opportunity to measure functionality and general symptoms at different levels. Drawing from the existing litera-

Table 3.1
Functionality and general symptoms at five different levels

Level	Description	Example
1	'Bare' functionality and general symptoms	Mobility with two paralysed legs Vision with no glasses, contact lenses, or laser surgery
2	With medical technologies	Surgery Gene therapy Behavioural counselling Medication Pacemaker
3	With non-human aids	Glasses Contact lenses Hearing aid Wheelchair Artificial arms
4	With human assistance	Human attendant
5	With accommodating environmental factors	Barrier-free physical environment Newspapers with large fonts

ture,[9] I identify five levels of functionality and general symptoms (see table 3.1).

The first level is 'bare' functionality and general symptoms, which involves no medical technologies and non-human aids. The 'bare' vision of a short-sighted person, for example, is the vision level without glasses. After becoming a victim of a landmine, Mai's 'bare' mobility is her mobility with two paralysed legs.

The second level is functionality and general symptoms with medical technologies, which aims at physiological changes (Salomon et al. 2003). I use the term 'medical technologies' broadly, to include such medical interventions as surgery, gene therapy, behavioural counselling, and medication, and such medical devices as a pacemaker. Should one focus on this level of functionality, one would measure, for example, the vision level of a short-sighted person after laser surgery, and the functionality of a person with HIV receiving antiretrovirals. In Mai's case, nowhere are medical technologies currently available to regenerate a lost arm or revive paralysed legs.

The third level is functionality and general symptoms with non-human aids. Non-human aids do not change human physiology but aim to improve functionality and general symptoms (Salomon et al. 2003). Examples of non-human aids include glasses, a hearing aid, a wheelchair, and artificial arms. Mai's functionality in Japan and the United States at this level is her functionality with an artificial arm and a wheelchair.

The fourth level is functionality and general symptoms with human assistance. Human assistance is the help of another person provided either informally (e.g., by family members) or formally (e.g., by a personal care attendant service). Access to human assistance depends both on individual and societal resources. In addition, such non-material factors as societal support, acceptance, culture, and tradition affect the use of human assistance. In Cambodia, Mai could not afford human assistance primarily due to the lack of resources of her family and society. The lack of human assistance to her in Japan, on the other hand, had more to do with the social acceptance of people with disabilities than the lack of resources.

Finally, the fifth level of functionality and general symptoms includes accommodating environmental factors. Similar to human assistance, accommodating environmental factors depend on the resources and non-material factors of a society. A near-sighted person, for example, could read newspapers printed in large fonts without glasses. Mai could move around more widely in the United States than Japan because of the barrier-free physical environment in the States.

Using the model above, one can summarize Mai's health as follows. After becoming a victim of a landmine, her 'bare' functionality and general symptoms in Cambodia, Japan, and the United States were the same. No medical technologies existed in any of these three countries that could change her physiology. Non-human aids improved her health in Japan. Human assistance and accommodating environmental factors further improved her health in the United States.

Which level of functionality and general symptoms should health status measures assess? Should they assess only 'bare' functionality and general symptoms (level 1)? Or should they assess functionality and general symptoms with medical technologies (level 2), non-human aids (level 3), and human assistance (level 4)? Should health status measures also pay attention to environmental factors specific to the person being assessed (level 5)?

EXISTING HEALTH STATUS MEASURES AND
DIFFERENT LEVELS OF HEALTH

In this section I look at how existing health status measures deal with different levels of functionality and general symptoms. I use two examples

of health status measures: the Health Utilities Index Mark 3 (hereafter
called the HUI) and the health status measure in the World Health
Survey (hereafter called the WHS). It is not my intention to provide a systematic review of existing health status measures. I selected these two
measures as pioneers that explicitly acknowledge, and provide conceptual discussion of, different levels of functionality and general symptoms.

The HUI. The HUI assesses eight dimensions of functionality and
general symptoms: vision, hearing, speech, ambulation, dexterity,
emotion, cognition, and pain (Feeny et al. 1995, 494–5). According to
its developers, the HUI aims to measure 'within-the-skin' experiences
and to separate health from any assessment of social interaction (Feeny
et al. 1995, 491). The concept of the 'within-the-skin' experiences
derives from the work by Ware and his colleagues, who explain it thus:
'In a model of health status at an individual level, physical and mental variables are similar in that they "end at the skin." They do not
directly involve other people or factors outside the individual. By contrast, social functioning extends the concept of health beyond the individual to include the quantity and quality of social contacts and social
resources' (Ware et al. 1981, 621). Although 'within-the-skin' and 'end
at the skin' possess slightly different connotations, following the
description by Ware and his colleagues, the dividing line is between
level 3 and level 4 in the model above. 'Bare' health (level 1) with
medical technologies (level 2) and non-human aids (level 3) are within
the assessment of health, while human assistance (level 4) and accommodating environmental factors (level 5) are not.

How does the HUI questionnaire reflect the concept proposed by
Ware and his colleagues? The HUI questionnaire does not ask about the
use of medical technologies, by implication presuming their inclusion
in the questions. Compatible with the concept by Ware and his colleagues, the HUI questionnaire explicitly asks questions about the use
of non-human aids (for example, glasses and contact lenses in vision,
hearing aids in hearing, walking equipment and wheelchairs in ambulation, and special tools in dexterity) and assesses health states with
these non-human aids. The HUI questionnaire also asks questions
about the use of human assistance (for example, in ambulation and
dexterity). Inconsistent with the concept of Ware and his colleagues,
it includes states of health with human assistance in the assessment
of health. The HUI questionnaire does not ask about environmental
factors.

Table 3.2
The Health Utilities Index (HUI) Mark 3 vision scoring system

Level	Single-Attribute HRQL Score	Description
1	1	Able to see well enough to read ordinary newsprint and recognize a friend on the other side of the street, without glasses or contact lenses.
2	0.95	Able to see well enough to read ordinary newsprint and recognize a friend on the other side of the street, but with glasses.
3	0.73	Able to read ordinary newsprint with or without glasses but unable to recognize a friend on the other side of the street, even with glasses.
4	0.59	Able to recognize a friend on the other side of the street with or without glasses but unable to read ordinary newsprint, even with glasses.
5	0.38	Unable to read ordinary newsprint and unable to recognize a friend on the other side of the street, even with glasses.
6	0	Unable to see at all.

Source: Feeny et al. (2000).

The HUI scoring system penalizes the use of a non-human aid in all four dimensions that acknowledge non-human aids. A concrete example illustrates this point. Table 3.2 lists levels of vision and corresponding health-related quality of life (HRQL) scores (single-attribute) in the HUI.[10] As table 3.2 shows, the HUI assigns a lower score for someone who is able to see well enough to read ordinary newsprint and recognize a friend on the other side of the street with glasses (0.95, level 2) than for someone who can do so without glasses or contact lenses (1.0, level 1).

How does the HUI measure the ambulation level of Mai as a landmine survivor? Because the ambulation dimension in the HUI is specifically about walking, Mai's ambulation level would consistently be level 6, cannot walk at all, in Cambodia, Japan, and the United States.

The WHS. The WHS assesses dimensions of mobility, self-care, pain, cognition, interpersonal activities, vision, sleep and energy, and affect

(World Health Organization 2000b). The WHS bases its concept on the International Classification of Functioning, Disability, and Health (ICF) (Salomon et al. 2003; World Health Organization 2001). The WHO researchers provide insightful discussion regarding different levels of functionality and general symptoms (Salomon et al. 2003). They argue that the distinction between medical technologies and non-human aids is 'inappropriate,' because such a distinction 'would omit many health system interventions that are commonly perceived to improve health': 'The distinction we propose here leaves us with personal interventions (drugs, implanted devices, external devices and aids) that improve capacity in a health domain and are available to individuals in the wide range of environments that they are likely to encounter, i.e., interventions that are essentially within individual control rather than environmentally determined' (Salomon et al. 2003, 305). As to the environmental factors, 'in the interest of comparability' the WHO researchers opted to assess health states by 'a single global standard' rather than the environment within which a respondent lives (Salomon et al. 2003, 305).

As in the HUI, the distinction dividing the measurement boundary is level three and four in the aforementioned model. However, the WHS questionnaire does not ask about medical technologies. The only non-human aids mentioned in the WHS questionnaire are glasses and contact lenses in the vision dimension. It is unclear how the WHS questionnaire reflects the concepts of human assistance and environmental factors. The WHS does not specifically ask about human assistance in each dimension, but at the beginning of the questionnaire the WHS asks: 'please answer this question taking into account any assistance you have available' (World Health Organization 2000b). The WHS does not explicitly mention environmental factors, but at the beginning of the questionnaire the following qualification appears: 'while doing the activity in the *way that you usually do it*' (World Health Organization 2000b, original emphasis).

The WHS score is currently under development and is not yet available (Salomon et al. 2004). Judging from the questionnaire, unlike the HUI, the WHS does not penalize the use of non-human aids. Questions in the vision dimension proceed as in table 3.3. The WHS first identifies the use of glasses or contact lenses. It then asks the same question about vision regardless of the use of glasses or contact lenses. The WHS treat users and non-users of glasses and contact lenses identically. Based on the intended concept and construct of WHS, Mai's mobility would be

Table 3.3
Health status descriptions, vision, World Health Survey

Do you wear *glasses or contact lenses*?

(If respondent says YES to this question, preface the next 2 questions with 'Please answer the following questions taking into account your glasses or contact lenses.')

1. Yes
2. No

In the last 30 days, how much difficulty did you have in seeing and recognizing *a person you know across the road* (i.e., from a distance of about 20 metres)?

1. None
2. Mild
3. Moderate
4. Severe
5. Extreme / Cannot do

Source: World Health Organization (2000).

worse in Cambodia than in Japan and the United States, but the same in Japan and the United States.

IMPLICATIONS FOR HEALTH STATUS MEASURES

Why should we be concerned about different levels of functionality and general symptoms in the construction and application of health status measures? Mai's case demonstrates that the assessment of the same functionality and general symptoms differs depending on the level one looks at. When health status survey questions are ambiguous about which level of functionality or general symptoms they are enquiring into, the decision on the inclusion of medical technologies, non-human aids, human assistance, and environmental factors in the assessment of health is inevitably left to the respondents. Just looking at answers, researchers would not know what factors respondents decided to include or exclude. Even using the same health status survey, then, researchers may, without recognizing it, be assessing 'bare' health at one time and 'bare' health with aids or assistance at another time. The preceding discussion, at the very least, suggests that researchers need to decide what they want to measure and develop a health status measure that reflects their decision.

The HUI and the WHS are examples of health status measures that explicitly acknowledge different levels of functionality and general symptoms. Yet, neither of them applies their chosen concepts consistently to their health status questionnaires. For example, the HUI's concept of separating health from the assessment of social interaction does not support the inclusion of human assistance in the assessment of ambulation and dexterity. The WHS questionnaire only mentions glasses and contact lenses as non-human aids, whereas the HUI also mentions walking equipment and wheelchairs in the mobility dimension. Neither the HUI nor the WHS explicitly asks about the use of medical technologies. Can one always assume that respondents of the HUI and WHS surveys assess their health taking into account, for example, their use of medication or a pacemaker?

Even if the questionnaires perfectly reflected the chosen concepts, the HUI and the WHS would assess the health of the same person differently. Mai's mobility level, for example, would be different according to the HUI and the WHS due to different definitions of mobility. The HUI asks about walking, while the WHS asks about moving around. Researchers using a health status measure should pay attention to how the questionnaire reflects the chosen concept.

WHAT SHOULD HEALTH STATUS MEASURES ASSESS?

Both the HUI and the WHS agree that the assessment of health should include medical technologies and non-human aids. The boundary that the HUI and the WHS set out is the individual. Things that can be within a person or move with a person are within the assessment of health.

I agree with their decision on setting the boundary at the individual for two reasons. First, the focus on the individual maintains a unique feature of health, that is, that each individual has a distinct health experience. Second, the focus on the individual is appropriate in the light of a widely shared understanding of health: health as a multipurpose resource useful for any life plan. Health as a resource belongs to a person. If we were to include social interactions in health measurement, our concern about health as a resource belonging to an individual would be lost. In addition, health as a basic, multi-purpose resource implies universality. Thus, as the WHS researchers argue (Salomon et al. 2003, 305), one should assume functionality and general symptoms in the standardized environment rather than a specific environment in which a respondent is living.[11]

One possible objection to the inclusion of medical technologies and non-human aids in the assessment of health is that they may jeopardize international or longitudinal comparison of health states. If two populations were vastly different in terms of medical and technological development, the availability of medical technologies and non-human aids could greatly affect the assessment of health states. Is this a problem? I think not. Even basic health statistics, such as life expectancy and infant mortality, are not free from medical and technological development. We do not adjust these basic health statistics for the level of medical and technological development of countries where we obtain the statistics. Similarly, we do not need to worry about the effect of the medical and technological development on health states. The availability of medical technologies and non-human aids is part of the determinants of functionality and general symptoms.

Setting the boundary between levels 3 and 4, how best can researchers construct health status measures? It is beyond the scope of this book to give a full account of the construction of health status measures. Here I discuss only two issues. First, an ideal health status measure would be decomposable by medical technologies and non-human aids. For example, a decomposable health status measure would not only assess the vision of the short-sighted after laser surgery or with glasses or contact lenses but also identify how much of the vision is attributable to laser surgery, glasses, or contact lenses (figure 3.4). An ideal questionnaire would then ask questions about functionality and general symptoms with and without medical technologies and non-human aids, and identify what medical technologies and non-human aids a respondent uses. The practicality of this proposal needs further examination. Nonetheless, decomposition is attractive because in a world of limited resources we would be interested in knowing how a certain level of functionality and general symptoms are realized and at what cost.

The second issue relates to the scoring system of health status measures. Should a health status measure assign the same score for the same function level regardless of the use of medical technologies or non-human aids? The WHS does so, but the HUI does not. I support the WHS's procedure.

Recall that the HUI penalizes the use of non-human aids. The HRQL score for someone with good vision without laser surgery, glasses, or contact lenses is 1.0 (see table 3.2). Assuming laser surgery as a 'within-the-skin' experience, the HRQL score for someone with the same good vision after laser surgery would also be 1.0. However, the HRQL score

Figure 3.4   Assessment of the vision of the short-sighted

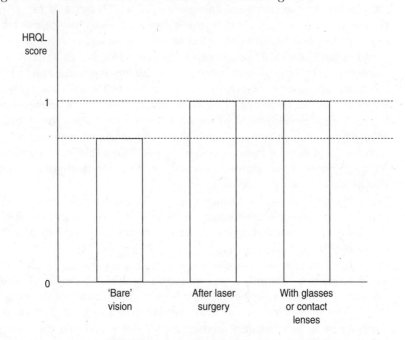

A short-sighted person can improve his or her vision by laser surgery or using eyeglasses or contact lenses. An ideal health state measure would be able to identify how much improvement is attributable to laser surgery, glasses, or contact lenses, and give the same score for the same improvement brought about by medical technology (in this example, laser surgery) and non-human aids (in this example, glasses, or contact lenses).

for a user of glasses or contact lenses with the same good vision would be 0.95.

By penalizing the use of non-human aids, the HUI implies that 'bare' health and 'bare' health with medical technologies are equally good and are better than 'bare' health with non-human aids. A reason for the penalty may be that one can lose, forget, or break non-human aids. However, we do not always prefer medical technologies to non-human aids to improve functionality or general symptoms. Despite the availability of laser surgery, for example, most people rely on glasses or contact lenses to improve vision. The wider use of glasses or contact lenses reflects consideration of such various factors as safety, effectiveness, cost, and convenience.

One way to investigate the best way to improve health is to conduct a cost-effectiveness analysis. To do so, we need to assess the effectiveness using the same scale for all alternatives as figure 3.4 illustrates. With the HUI in the current form, it is difficult to conduct a fair cost-effectiveness analysis for medical technologies and non-human aids.

My analysis above has one important limitation: I treated similarly all different dimensions of functionality and general symptoms in my discussion. Mai, to illustrate my points, has obvious disabilities. Can the argument be extended to less obvious disabilities, for example, problems in cognitive function? Further exploration of issues of medical technologies, aids, assistance, and environmental factors may require different assessment for different dimensions of functionality and general symptoms.

The issues explored in here are complex, but, I believe, necessary considerations for the further development of measuring health and health equity.

FIVE-CATEGORY SELF-PERCEIVED HEALTH
The model I offered above is also useful for examining the use of five-category self-perceived health, a very popular health measure in health inequity analysis. A person's self-perceived health is assessed by such a question as follows: Would you say your health in general is excellent, very good, good, fair, or poor? The way question and answer are phrased varies, but the answer is usually in these five categories. This is one of the standard questions in health surveys elsewhere in the world.[12]

Self-perceived health can be understood as the health that each individual perceives influenced by all factors discussed above – 'bare' health experiences, use of non-human aids and human assistance, wealth, culture, tradition, social support, and acceptance – as well as one's personality. The appropriateness of the use of self-perceived health as a health status measure can be examined by the question of why we value health. If health were to be measured by self-perceived health, in an extreme case, it would be possible to raise people's health status by making them more optimistic despite low levels of 'bare' health experiences or the lack of availability of non-human aids and human assistance. Can poor health experience be substituted by optimism? Does a health experience with no substitution of optimism reflect the same level of health-related welfare or the same use of health as a multipurpose resource? If it did, there would not be much reason to be concerned about health to begin with. There are some reports on agreement between self-perceived health and more 'objective' measures assessed by health professionals or physical tests (Idler and Kasl 1995; Okun et al. 1984), but not always (Sen 2002). Five-category self-perceived health no doubt provides rich information unavailable otherwise, but relying on it exclusively would be misleading.

3.3 Unit of Time

Health is a lifelong experience. The process of health production that we have discussed above might appear to be static, as we have not so far paid attention to the dynamics of time in our analyses of health, its determinants, and their distributions. In reality, our health status changes over time, each age presenting various sensitivities to different health determinants. Each health determinant makes a unique contribution to our health at different times in our lives. These issues about time are perhaps among the most challenging areas in understanding health.

The issue of time also arises in general philosophical discussion of equality: within what period of time should we seek equity? This question is frequently deferred, the entire lifetime often assumed to be an appropriate egalitarian unit of time (McKerlie 1992, 277nn1–2). Some, albeit few, philosophers challenge this general assumption (Daniels 1988; McKerlie 1989; Temkin 1993, chap. 8) and suggest that whatever equity perspective one might choose, the question of equity and time has independent importance. Learning from their discussion, and paying attention to the dynamics of time in health production, in this section we examine what might be an appropriate time unit in conceptualizing and measuring health equity.

McKerlie proposes that there are at least three different time frames within which we seek equity (1989). His classification is directly applicable to the health context, and figures 3.5 and 3.6 introduce them accordingly. Suppose that human life consists only of three stages, roughly thirty years each: the young, the adult, and the old. Now we have four birth cohorts born every thirty years, A, B, C, and D. Although I use the term 'birth cohort,' in my usage this means merely a group of people who experience different stages of life in the same calendar years. It thus does not imply any specific characteristics of a certain period of time, for example, the technological developments and cultural norms that a specific birth cohort collectively experiences.

Figure 3.5 illustrates the stages of life each of the four birth cohorts passes through in calendar years from 1900 to 2050. Now imagine that we had survey data available for health equity analysis for 1960 and 1990. We are primarily interested in health equity in 1990, and how it has changed since 1960.

Applying McKerlie's classification, there are at least three ways to measure health equity in 1990 and compare it to that of 1960 (figure 3.6). The first is the whole-life approach, in which we measure the overall health experience in the lifetime of an individual or a group of people and assess their inequity. As figure 3.6 illustrates, the whole-life approach might measure health expectations, instead of outcomes, of the birth cohort D: what are the expected health experiences of those who are born in the survey year, 1990? The birth cohort D would consist of different groups of people, each of them would present different health expectations. Based on a chosen perspective on health equity, we would measure inequity in the whole-life health expectations. Anyone who did not like to use health expectations could use health outcomes instead. The point here is not whether we use health expectations or outcomes or even determinants, but rather how we measure the health experiences of, as McKerlie says, a 'complete life' (1989).

The second approach is a familiar cross-sectional measurement in empirical health research. We take a snapshot of the health experiences of people alive in 1990 all together, irrespective of their life stages. McKerlie calls this approach the 'simultaneous segments view' (1989).

The third approach is the life-stage approach. It is still a snapshot, cross-sectional measurement, but this time we pay attention to the different life stages people experience in 1990. That is, we measure health equity within each of the young, the adult, and the old. When we compare health inequity in 1960 and 1990, we compare health inequity among the young, the adult, and the old in 1960 and 1990 separately. McKerlie calls this third approach the 'corresponding segment views' (1989).

Which of these three approaches might be the most appropriate time unit in health equity analysis? This question can be best examined by going back to our understanding of why we value health. Recall the view of health as a multi-purpose good. In this understanding of health, health is a multi-purpose resource that enables us to do things we value and to seek good lives whatever our conceptions of a good life. Health, in other words, is a resource that enhances opportunities in life, and it is reasonable to think that we appreciate the opportunities that health

Figure 3.5 Birth cohorts and calendar years

Birth cohort	Calendar year					
	1900	1930	1960	1990	2020	2050
A	Young	Adult	Old			
B		Young	Adult	Old		
C			Young	Adult	Old	
D				Young	Adult	Old

Figure 3.6 Three types of unit of time

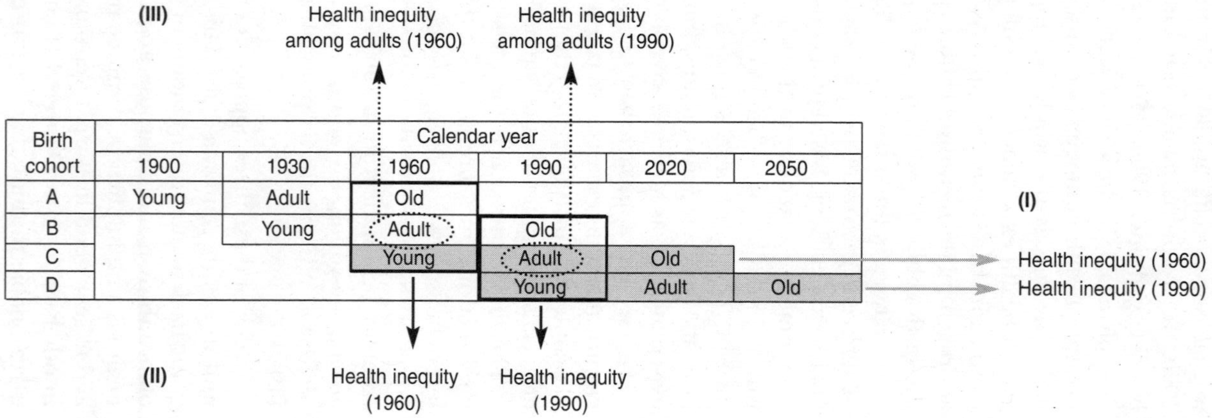

(III) Health inequity among adults (1960)   Health inequity among adults (1990)

Birth cohort	Calendar year					
	1900	1930	1960	1990	2020	2050
A	Young	Adult	Old			
B		Young	Adult	Old		
C			Young	Adult	Old	
D				Young	Adult	Old

Health inequity (1960)   Health inequity (1990)

(I) Health inequity (1960)   Health inequity (1990)

brings differently at different stages of life. The same good health, for example, may bring more opportunities to someone's life in their twenties than in their seventies. It also seems reasonable to assume that we appreciate different kinds of opportunities in different stages of life. Mobility may be valued more in childhood than in old adulthood, for example. As empirical studies show, furthermore, good health in earlier life stages is in itself an opportunity for good health in later life stages (Kawachi, Subramanian, and Almeida-Filho 2002; Power, Matthews, and Manor 1998).

To simplify the discussion, in the example of figures 3.5 and 3.6, I suggested only three life stages: the young, the adult, and the old. Researchers actually suggest many different ways to partition the life cycle. Yet they share a similar understanding of the basic health experiences of human beings. Understanding this shared view helps us see why we might pay attention to life stages in health equity analysis.

Hertzman and his colleagues, for example, propose four stages of the life cycle: perinatal (preterm to 1 year), misadventure (1–44 years), chronic disease (45–74 years), and senescence (75 years and older), each of which represents different health risks (1994). Even in developed countries, the perinatal period still presents high health risks, and survival of this period is considered to be so important that it is often used as an indicator of population health. Once babies survive this period, what comes next is the misadventure period, when major health risks are not diseases but accidents, violence, and suicide. When people enter their mid-forties, chronic diseases begin to appear as principal health concerns. For those who survive this period, the subsequent period is considered to be a more or less successful process of aging and dying. There will be further debate on the precise division of life stages, but whatever it may be, it should reflect the general development of a person as well as health risks and vulnerability, for example, the perinatal period, childhood, adolescent, young adulthood, old adulthood, and 'old old.'

According to the whole-life approach, what matters is the overall health experience. It does not take into account that health is generally strongly correlated with age and that the importance of opportunity that health brings might vary at different life stages. The whole-life approach misses important information.

Similarly, the familiar cross-sectional snapshot of health equity, the simultaneous segments view, seems to be too crude – it does not pay attention to how age is distributed within a population in health inequity analysis. Figure 3.6 might give the impression that the age compositions of the 1960 and 1990 populations are roughly the same, but this is not often the case in real life. Suppose that the 1960 and 1990 populations did differ in terms of the size of age groups, that is, the frail old was proportionally much bigger in the 1990 than the 1960 population. Suppose further that because of this difference in demography, we observed a greater health inequality in 1990 than 1960. Is this inequality inequitable?

In the understanding of health as a multi-purpose resource enhancing opportunities in our lives, Norman Daniels does not see health inequality between the young and the old as inequitable (1988).[13] Although we try to prolong living years and postpone the decline of health-adjusted quality of life, we all must die sometime, and health-adjusted quality of life tends to deteriorate towards death. Daniels importantly points out that such a biological ageing process is what everyone experiences (1988, 41). This is why, he continues, unlike discrimination based on race or ethnicity – circumstances that, once we are born, we cannot change – the fact that the old are generally less healthy than the young is not a concern for inequity. Consequently, according to this view, some sort of age adjustment would be necessary in order for the simultaneous segments view to provide meaningful health equity information. Of course, the crude assessment is useful in the same way as any crude epidemiological assessment is, but that should be just the start of an analytic plan.[14]

From the preceding discussion, in the understanding of health as a resource, the life-stage approach seems to provide the most appropriate time unit when thinking about health equity. An obvious problem of the life-stage approach – also familiar in the field of the summary measure of population health – is the neglect of health experience of the past and the future. This leads to two major consequences. First of all, in the life-stage approach we must think about how to deal with the dead. The whole-life approach by definition includes death as the end point of a whole life and the issue of the inclusion of the dead in health inequity analysis does not arise. But this is not the case for the life-stage approach – someone who died in adulthood would simply disappear in old age, for example. Recognizing death as a health outcome, or more precisely in our context as the complete exhaustion of health as a resource, one might argue that counting the living only provides partial information concerning health inequity. However healthy the living population may be, if it was coupled with the deaths from among the vast majority of the population, we may not be able to capture the state of health inequity merely by looking at the health of the living. The life-stage approach must find a way to include the dead in health inequity analysis.

Another consequence of focusing independently on a particular life stage is that we cannot assess health inequity over the entire life period. This is because we are not yet sure about how to value health at different life stages and combine it as the whole-life experience. The ideal approach regarding the unit of time in health inequity analysis might be a compromise between the life stage and whole-life approach (McKerlie 1989; Temkin 1993, chap. 8), but for that we need further discussion on a different weight for a different life stage reflecting our relative value of each life stage. Some proposals have actually been suggested for assessing the effect of age weight on health, most notably, the WHO's age weight in the construction of DALYs or Disability-Adjusted Life Years (Murray 1996, 54–61). But the issue has not been settled. Until a general consensus is obtained, the life stage-approach appears to be the best option. The life-stage approach reflects our fundamental value of health while leaving the unsettled issues open. Furthermore, support for the life-stage approach comes from the understanding of health as a multi-purpose resource, which is a foundation of many of the equity perspectives we looked at in chapter 2. This suggests that any perspectives on health equity that regard health as a multi-purpose resource should assess health equity at different life stages. Empirically, this means that we stratify a population by age group and measure health inequity within each age group.

3.4 Unit of Analysis

Health inequity has most often been documented as differences in average health between groups. Researchers use such characteristics as education, income, occupation, race or ethnicity, and geographic location to divide people into groups. Given the dominance of the group approach, measuring health inequity across individuals has been rare. However, Gakidou, Murray, and Frenk renewed interest in measuring health inequity across individuals in *The World Health Report 2000*. Since then, there has been a heated debate over whether health inequity would be better analysed by group or individual. In this section, we discuss in what way the group and individual approaches differ in conceptualizing and measuring health inequity.[15]

Before proceeding, clarification is in order with regard to the usage of 'group' or 'grouping' below. In empirical health research, we group data in various ways. One way is stratification, which applies to the age groups discussed in the previous section. Stratifying by age groups, we examine health inequity within each age group. Grouping in the context of the unit of analysis is different. We divide individuals into groups using a certain characteristic. In health inequity analysis, we usually compare the average of each group. In short, stratification directs us to health inequity within a group, whereas grouping as the unit of analysis generally turns our attention to health inequity between groups.

It might seem attractive to think that the central characteristic that divides the two approaches is the presence of a normative stand (Murray, Gakidou, and Frenk 1999). The group approach, in this view, is only concerned about health inequalities caused by certain factors, most notably socio-economic, and the choice of group characteristics prescribes what is just or unjust, equitable or inequitable. The individual approach, on the other hand, distinguishes the process of measuring health inequality from that of judging when health inequalities are unfair, unjust, or inequitable, and determining why. The individual approach, so this view goes, measures health inequalities whatever their causes and leaves the decision about which theory of justice is most appropriate for judging whether the health distribution is inequitable to those using the information.

This value-free claim is misleading. Most of all, it confuses non-moral and moral interests in health inequality. As we discussed at the very beginning of the introduction, one might simply be interested in describing the phenomenon of health inequality and investigating its mechanism. For such non-moral interest in health distribution, measuring across individuals would probably be best, given the general assumption that individual data, rather than aggregate data, can better reveal true associations. But if one wished to measure health distribution for ethical reasons, that is, to measure health inequity, whether measuring it across individuals or groups, one would already betray a normative interest.

This value-free claim also misjudges the role normative positions can play in scientific endeavours. Although it is undesirable to let norms and values colour an investigation, they play a necessary part in deciding what questions to ask. What phenomena we are interested in and what aspects of them we feel are particularly important is a function of our total world view, which includes our normative views. The group theorist is using her beliefs about what aspects of health inequality are of moral importance to decide what questions to ask about the inequality. This does not, however, hinder the investigation itself from being in compliance with the demands of the scientific method.

Value judgments, furthermore, enter at various stages when one is measuring health inequity. As we discussed in previous sections of this chapter, once we consider the moral reason to be interested in the distribution of health, many measurement decisions depend on more than data availability or analytic convenience. The decision about what aspect of health we should focus on, for example, would not merely be determined by what health variable is available but why we value health as a distribution good.

As we examined in chapter 2, there are various ways to define which health inequalities are inequitable. It is a mistake to think that measuring health inequity across individuals lets users of the information to define health equity. The health inequity concept proposed by Gakidou, Murray, and Frenk, for example, with which health inequity is measured across individuals, does look at health inequality determined by certain causes. Take another example from chapter 2. In the view of health equity as satisfying the minimally adequate level of health, we might want to apply this principle to each individual in society. We would then, according to this view, measure health inequity across individuals, but this is hardly value-free. One can hold a certain normative view in mind regarding what makes a health distribution inequitable and still measure it across individuals. It is not only the group approach that prescribes a certain normative stand in health inequity analysis; the individual approach does so too.[16]

If the central characteristic that divides the individual and group approach is not the presence or absence of a normative stand, what is it that separates these two approaches? How might we choose one from the other? Below I discuss three key arguments that distinguish the individual and group approach.

Among Whom Do We Want to Seek Health Equity?

The first and most fundamental question dividing the two approaches is that of among whom we would like to seek health equity. Some people say across groups in the belief that some group characteristics cannot morally justify observing health inequality. For example, we might think that differences in functionality can be justified between the young and old but not between Black and White people. By looking at inequalities between groups, we may 'uncover those inequalities in health that we regard as particularly unjust' (Anand 2002, 487). A popular group characteristic used is socio-economic status (SES). This captures our intuition that health should not be determined by or even simply associated with the general socio-economic power of a person represented by their education, income, or occupation. In chapter 2, we discussed how Rawls's theory of justice and fairness and Walzer's view of inequity as dominance might support this intuition.

SES is not the only group characteristic used in health inequity analysis. The International Society for Equity in Health (ISEqH), for example, defines health equity as 'the absence of systematic differences in one or more aspects of health status across socially, demographically, or geographically defined population groups' (Starfield 2002, 452). Also, the second goal of *Healthy People 2010* is 'to eliminate health disparities among segments of the population, including differences that occur by gender, race or ethnicity, education or income, disability, geographic location, or sexual orientation' (U.S. Department of Health and Human Services 2000). The primary reason to choose a certain group characteristic in health inequity analysis would be based on the assumption that no health inequality observed across groups divided by the chosen characteristic can be morally justified. The ISEqH's and *Healthy People 2010*'s views expand such group characteristics much more than SES. Selecting a reasonable group characteristic is a difficult task, and this exercise leads us back to the question of which health inequality is inequitable.

Both the ISEqH and *Healthy People 2010*, for example, regard geographic location as a group characteristic that cannot morally justify an observed health inequality. Geographically defined population groups can reflect such social or political issues as systematic differences of general social conditions between rural and urban areas. But they can also reflect factors closely related to nature, for example, climate. If a tropical region in a country has people with low health status due to a very high prevalence of malaria but a temperate region in that same country does not, and the high prevalence of malaria does not reflect socio-economic conditions but only climate, is this difference inequitable? Both of these two views would say yes, but is this reasonable?

As this example suggests, the question of which group characteristic makes sense in health inequity analysis directly relates to the question of which health distributions are inequitable. This point deserves more serious attention than it usually receives. In addition, what is even more difficult to decide is which group characteristic might be morally more important than another in seeking health equity. Unless one has ideological interests in a specific group, answering this question requires a comprehensive theory of justice.

Seeking equity across groups is often taken for granted in health equity policy. But in general philosophical discussion of equality, there is a counter-argument: what we are concerned with is not equity between groups themselves but equity between members of groups (Temkin 1993, chap. 4). While the individual approach uses the most disaggregated unit of analysis, that is, the individual, the group approach usually compares representative characteristics of groups, that is, group averages, which mask within-group individual characteristics. There would be less concern if all members of a group were clearly separated from all members of other groups in terms of health, but this is unlikely to be the case. Moreover, reducing inequality between groups does not always coincide with reducing inequality within groups or reducing total inequality within the overall population. Can those who support the group approach invariably justify the focus on health inequality between groups classified with a particular characteristic regardless of other types of inequity? The focus on group averages could mislead our attention based on group classification we prescribe.

There is also a classic political argument supporting equity across individuals: we should develop a society in which an individual is considered only as an individual irrespective of any group affiliation (Young 2001). On this view, the use of the group classification itself supports discrimination and encourages divisiveness, however trivially. The opponents of affirmative action often use this argument. Although this view is not clearly pronounced with regard to health inequity, as a fundamental political stance it has force.

Comparability of Health Inequity Analysis

The ease of comparison of the individual approach has been mentioned as a methodological advantage (Illsley and Le Grand 1987; Murray, Gakidou, and Frenk 1999). An unlimited number of group choices are possible, and group definitions vary. Different populations prefer different groupings, for example, income in the United States and occupation in Europe, to represent a general position in the socio-economic hierarchy. Studies understandably adopt different groupings

or group definitions reflecting the political, philosophical, and sociological concerns of the particular environment within which these
equity studies are conducted. It is argued, however, that a disadvantage
of the group approach is its inability to compare inequalities between
populations as well as within a population at different times (Valkonen
1993).

The individual is the ultimate and most robust unit of analysis. The
comparability of the individual approach is certainly an attractive
feature, but a group choice might not be as much of a problem as it first
appears. Such factors as income, education, and occupation are often
used as a proxy for SES. But what exactly is the SES we are interested in?
A full discussion of this point is beyond the scope of this book, but a
brief discussion is relevant. Inspired by Marilyn Frye's analogy, Iris
Young provides a helpful insight about what we might after all want to
capture by various grouping in health inequality analyses (Young 2001).
Frye uses the metaphor of a birdcage (1983). She invites us to imagine
a bird confined in a cage. Suppose that the bird is the oppressed and
each cage wire is a factor that prevents her from being free, for
example, discriminatory treatment against women, or belonging to a
marginalized racial or ethnic group or having low income and education. If we focus only on one cage wire, we cannot see that the bird is
caged. Only when we sit back and see all the wires together does the
cage that confines the bird appear before our eyes. Young rephrases this
metaphor as structural inequalities. I believe the kind of inequity in
health that we try to capture by various grouping of SES is structural
inequality in Young's term. One group characteristic, she says, would
not allow us to say much about the kind of inequality we hope to understand; nonetheless, that is an important step towards our goal.

When we have a specific concern for health between particular socio-
economic groups, investigating health inequity by that specific group
characteristic will provide immediate and important information.
Racial disparity in various social settings, for example, is a historical and
political concern in the United States and South Africa (McIntyre and
Gilson 2002; Thomas 2001). It is reasonable and perhaps even necessary
to consider racial disparity in health policy.

If, instead, structural inequity is the kind of inequity that the group
approach tries to measure, we should not rely merely on one socio-
economic variable (Muntaner 2002). We would wish to explore a way in
which we can systematically examine various socio-economic variables
in health inequity analysis. As much as we need to investigate more

about how each of these socio-economic factors affects health and how they relate to the others, we need a good understanding of what these group characteristics suggest in terms of justice. We reviewed some such attempts in chapter 2. These efforts are promising input to the field.

If the systematic investigation of a number of socio-economic factors is too ambitious, then we might try to find the best indicator for structural inequities. And different group characteristics might be the best indicators in different populations. If, for example, income reflected social strata in the United States and occupation in the United Kingdom, even though they are different variables, they are the best indicators of social strata. If this was the case, structural inequities in health would be comparable, even when social strata were measured differently in different populations. Gakidou, Murray, and Frenk are dismissive on this point, saying that we will never be able satisfactorily to come up with the best indicator of social strata as we will always find a new variable that produces contradictory health inequity results (Murray, Gakidou, and Frenk 1999, 540). But this comes from a misunderstanding of what the best indicator of social strata would be. It would not matter whether another variable leads to a different result as long as the indicator chosen best reflects social strata, which should be defined independently from its relationship to health.

The question of whether we can ever reasonably measure and compare structural inequities by one indicator needs to be examined through further discussion on what exactly we intend to measure by SES factors.

Selective Information by Averaging

The last key argument over the individual versus group approach is pragmatic. The group approach can neglect such a difficult problem as cost by averaging. In chapter 2 we discussed how society would go bankrupt if it adopted any of the perspectives on health equity introduced, except the view of health equity as health equality by SES and the view of health inequality as an indicator of general social justice. We might decide, for example, that society ought to help everyone who becomes ill due to factors beyond individual control or that it ought to help raise everyone's health level to the minimally adequate level of health. Among those whom society ought to help, there will always be the expensively and helplessly sick. If we selected the individual as the unit of health inequity analysis, we would face this problem head-on.

If, on the other hand, we chose a group as the unit of analysis, the troublesome cost problem would disappear. Say we support the view that society ought to help raise the average health level of each income group to a certain level of health. In each income group, we could expect that the expensively ill individual would be cancelled out by the healthy individual with no cost. The cost problem would disappear.

This selective information by averaging works not only for the cost issue but also for other purposes. The view of health inequity as inequality in health by SES, for example, conveniently masks individual variations by averaging within each socio-economic group. There may be risk lovers and misfortunes for which society does not have responsibility. If indeed the social structure has nothing to do with their distributions, they should be spread randomly across socio-economic groups, and their effects would not appear in comparing the average health of each socio-economic group. As we discussed in chapter 2, however, in the view of health inequity as inequality in health caused by factors beyond individual control, it is important to understand what is cancelled out and what is not by averaging.

Whether one regards the selective information by averaging as favourable convenience seems still debatable.

The three key arguments above for distinguishing the individual and group approach might give the impression that these are clear, dichotomous choices for the unit of analysis. From a quantitative methodological view, however, if we collected both individual and group data, we could examine health inequity across individuals as well as groups (Wolfson and Rowe 2001). This is presumably what Gakidou, Murray, and Frenk meant by constructing 'a better dependent variable' with the individual approach (Murray, Gakidou, and Frenk 1999).

In this joint approach, we can ask what proportion of the overall health inequality is due to a particular group characteristic and, among many group characteristics, which one contributes most to the overall health inequality. This means that the joint approach can help identify the most effective target in health equity policy. Those who support the group approach sometimes contend that only through it can we identify the target group for health equity policy and begin to explain causes and the mechanisms of health inequity.[17] But the conventional group approach examining a binary relationship can only hypothesize a target group or causal path, and the joint approach is necessary to see how effective that target might be.

The joint approach appears to be a promising strategy as it solves the weakness of both approaches. We will discuss it more in detail in chapter 4. It is worth emphasizing, however, that the joint approach cannot solve all problems, especially philosophical issues; the difficult philosophical problem of among whom health equity should be sought would still remain.

3.5 Different Perspectives on Health Equity Revisited

In this chapter, we looked at issues that need to be addressed upon transforming a health equity concept to a measurement strategy. How do they relate to the different perspectives on health equity discussed in chapter 2?

Measurement strategy in any analysis of health distribution always depends on data availability and technical convenience. In addition, this chapter emphasized that measurement decisions should always reflect research goals. If we are interested in a particular mechanism of health inequality, our chosen hypothesis ought to guide us towards the health variable we should use in the analysis. Similarly, if our primary interest in health inequality is its relationship to the mean health level of a population, we should measure the health inequality that has the greatest impact on the health of the overall population.

When we measure health distribution for moral concerns, our value of health as a distribution good should influence our measurement decisions on health, the unit of time, and the unit of analysis. Figure 3.7 summarizes which measurement strategies each perspective on health equity from chapter 2 is likely to endorse. Perspectives that consider health equity as equality in health, irrespective of the focus on a certain cause or level of health, would select function as the aspect of health and favour the life-stage approach as the desirable unit of time. These decisions reflect our fundamental value of health as a multi-purpose resource, which forms the basis of any of the perspectives that regard health equity as equality in health. In agreement with the developers of the HUI and the WHS, I argued that medical technologies and non-human aids should be included in the assessment of functionality and general symptoms. All five perspectives on health equity, except the perspective proposed by Gakidou, Murray, and Frenk, look at health outcome as the focal point of health equity. I pointed out that the focus on health expectation proposed by Gakidou, Murray, and Frenk is both conceptually and methodologically questionable.

Figure 3.7 Summary of chapter 3

Chapter 1	Chapter 2	Chapter 3				
		Health			Unit of time	Unit of analysis
Different reasons to be concerned about health inequality	Different perspectives on health inequity	Aspect	Expectation / outcome*	Medical technologies / aids / assistance / environmental factors		
Non-moral, non-ethical reasons	NA		As research goal directs			
Moral, ethical reasons — Utilitarian: health equality helps improve the overall population health	Utilitarian		As population health goal directs			
Egalitarian — Equity as equality in health — By socio-economic status		Function (capacity)	Outcome		Life stage	Group
By factors beyond individual control		Function (capacity)	Outcome		Life stage	Individual / group
By factors amenable to human interventions		Function (capacity)	Expectation**	Medical technologies & aids	Life stage	Individual**
Normal species functioning		Function (biological)	Outcome		Life stage	Individual
Capability approach		Function (capacity)	Outcome		Life stage	Individual
Health inequality as an indicator of social justice		Function (capacity)	Outcome		Life stage	Individual

* As discussed in the text, egalitarian perspectives aimed at equalizing determinants are possible. But here, I list only those that concern either expectation or outcome.

** In developing the WHO health inequality index, Gakidou, Murray, and Frenk (2000) attempted to measure inequity in health expectation across individuals, but as I discuss in the text, health expectation can only reasonably be measured for a group.

An important factor for selecting the unit of analysis is the question of among whom we wish to seek health equity. The view that considers health inequality caused by SES as inequitable would opt for the group as the unit of analysis. The view that regards health equity as satisfying the minimally adequate level of health, on the other hand, would favour the individual as the unit of analysis, because this view perceives health as something close to a right or an entitlement of every member of a society.

The other two perspectives do not seem to have a definitive answer to the question of among whom health equity should be sought. Their selection of the unit of analysis would depend on other considerations, that is, comparability and convenience from averaging. It is important to recognize which factors can be cancelled out by averaging and whether that procedure is compatible with the equity perspective adopted. Recall our discussion in chapter 2 on the view of inequity as inequality caused by factors beyond individual control. Looking at the average level of health in each socio-economic group is inappropriate for this perspective, as this strategy is bound to miss factors randomly distributed across socio-economic groups. Should one adopt this perspective and opt for the group as the unit of analysis, careful consideration would be necessary to determine which group characteristic to use and, with it, what factors to be cancelled out.

The perspective that treats health inequality as an indicator of social justice would make these measurement decisions differently from other perspectives. In this view, measurement decisions should reflect two interests, our value of health and health inequality as an information carrier of social justice. As in other perspectives, our value of health as a multi-purpose resource would direct this perspective to choose function with non-human aids as the aspect of health on which to focus and the life-stage approach for the unit of time. Since in this perspective we understand that how a society functions is expressed in health outcome, we would look at health outcome. Because this perspective intends to capture general social justice, the individual would be the favourable unit of analysis.

Having examined theories and key measurement strategies in this and previous chapters, we can now identify major challenges each perspective on health equity faces. The view of health inequity as inequality in health caused by SES has a good theoretical base owing to increasing attention from philosophers, and its selection of measurement strategies is straightforward. If one sought a theoretical base in Rawls's theory of justice as fairness, the major challenge of this perspective is which group characteristic to use. If one adopted Walzer's view of dominance as unjust, one would be free to examine different group characteristics. Walzer's view, moreover, can be easily transformed to an analytic plan of simply looking at correlations between health and other goods. While the straightforwardness is certainly an attraction, what Walzer's view ultimately suggests is social engineering, which goes much beyond the traditional health sector. Accordingly, it is unlikely to provide an immediate health policy implication.

Despite its intuitive appeal, the view of health inequity as health inequality caused by factors beyond individual control has many problems, both conceptually and methodologically. In chapter 2, we discussed how difficult it would be to define what exactly is under individual control. Even if we could come up with a reasonable definition, as Roemer's proposal suggests, empirically sorting out factors beyond individual control is challenging. As discussed above, it is not clear if the convenience of averaging by using the group as the unit of analysis works well with this perspective.

The health inequity perspective proposed by Gakidou, Murray, and Frenk, that is, inequity as inequality in health caused by factors amenable to human interventions, presents many problems due to its focus on health expectation. Health expectation does not reflect their intended equity concept, and estimating it for an individual is impractical. The immediate solution would be to look at inequality in health outcome across individuals. But, as in the case of the view of health inequity as health inequality caused by factors beyond individual control, sorting out desirable factors is challenging.

The view of health equity as satisfying the minimally adequate level of health has a good theoretical basis, and researchers can straightforwardly select measurement strategies. In this perspective, the connection between the health equity concept and measurement strategies is clear. Researchers in the empirical health sciences have not paid much attention to this perspective, but the application of this perspective to empirical analysis would show promise. Among the perspectives on health equity we have examined, only this view makes a strong theoretical support for measuring health inequity across individuals. The problems with this perspective are inherent in the theory itself. In chapter 2, we discussed three conceptual difficulties this perspective faces, defining the minimally adequate level of health, problems of cost, and the hopelessly sick.

Having examined measurement decisions from various aspects, we can think further about how the minimally adequate level of health in the normal species function view and the capability approach might be set. I showed in section 3.2 that the capability approach would focus on capacity as function, and function as health, whose minimally adequate level should be satisfied by every individual in society. I also discussed in section 3.3 that health inequity is best analysed within the same age group, which implies that the minimally adequate level of capacity would be defined in each age group. The minimally adequate level of capacity might then be defined simply as the average level of capacity in each age group. Setting the minimum level as the average is admittedly arbitrary, but we might think that the average level is what society can reasonably provide to its people, and taking the life-stage approach, the general biological ageing process of human species is accounted for. Similarly, we can set the minimally adequate level of function for the normal species functioning view, but this time, function is the biological construct and maintenance. In this case, the data on function would come from clinical examination rather than general health status questionnaires.

Lastly, the perspective of health inequality as an indicator of social justice also provides a plausible concept and straightforwardly selects measurement strategies. The theoretical base is shaky, but it expresses a reasonable account. Perhaps the biggest challenge of this perspective is, as in the case of Walzer's view of dominance as unjust, the lack of direct policy implications. Adopting this perspective, we would know the general level of social justice in a population, and this perspective provides an important reason why health inequality is in general bad. Yet, if we are to move on to policy-making in the pursuit of greater equity, we need further information and guidance.

To conclude this chapter, it is useful to clarify a question that some readers might have: why do I not discuss quality-adjusted life years (QALYs) and disability-adjusted life years (DALYs)? QALYs and DALYs belong to a family of health-adjusted life years (HALYs) that combines life years and quality of life related to health that goes with them. Using HALYs, we can say, for example, that my grandmother lived for ninety-three years but that the years she lived in full health, that is, HALYs, were eighty-five. Health status measures provide information on quality of life by ranking health states and assigning numerical values to each health state. Measuring health status is much more complicated than, say, measuring blood pressure, as it involves *evaluation* (Hausman 2006).

Key questions in measuring health status include (1) which aspects of health should we focus on? (2) how should we operationalize chosen aspects of health? and (3) how should we assign numerical values to different health states (Fryback 1998)? Among these three questions, (3) is arguably the most heated area of inquiry. For example, should we obtain preferences? If not, what would be an alternative? If so, whose preferences should we collect, those of experts, patients, or the general public? How should we then collect preferences, for example, using the Standard Gamble, the Time Trade-Off, or the visual analogue scale? Health status measures that assign numerical values to health states based on preferences are called health-related quality of life (HRQL) measures. HALYs whose quality of life information is obtained by health-related quality of life measures are QALYs. DALYs are a variant of QALYs, but DALYs use disability weight rather than health weight.[18]

The reasons why I do not discuss QALYs and DALYs in this book are twofold. First, in examining how to measure health, I started by asking what aspect of health we should consider *when we think of health equity*, and I defended function and general symptoms. Second, to the question of within what time frame we should seek health equity, I argued for the life-stage approach as opposed to the whole-life approach and the cross-sectional approach. If I had started by asking how we should measure health in general or if my conclusion for the second point had been the whole-life approach, I would have discussed QALYs and DALYs. Although health status measurement is in itself a fascinating research area and worth a book of its own, this book is about measuring health inequity, and our discussion on health status measures is accordingly necessarily limited.

4 How Can a Health Distribution Be Summarized into One Number?

4.1 Introduction

Chapters 1 and 2 helped us decide which health inequality we might explore for the assessment of health equity. Chapter 3 asked us what measurement choices might follow in transforming an equity concept to an empirical analysis. Together they should allow us to draw such health distributions as in figure 4.1.

The obvious next step in the assessment of health equity is to quantify the amount of health inequity such a health distribution as figure 4.1 presents. Note that the question of which health inequality is inequitable has already been taken care of by the time we can draw these health distributions, and they contain all the information that we judge to be inequitable or useful for the assessment of general social justice. More precisely, if we adopt the perspective of equity as equality in health, then we have already extracted desirable equity information from inequality through discussions in the previous chapters and are now contemplating how best to condense that equity information in a form easy to communicate. Similarly, if we opt for the view of health inequality as an indicator of social justice, then we have decided to pay attention to observing health inequality as a whole, and are now attempting to compress that information so as to quantitatively express the degree of health inequality as an indicator of social justice.

Traditionally, those who examine the dispersion of a distribution do not make a distinction between inequality and inequity, and they seem to assume that all information carried in a distribution is worthy of assessment. Their activity is usually called measurement of inequality,[1] and I follow this practice. Although the practice is to quantify equity

Figure 4.1 Health distributions

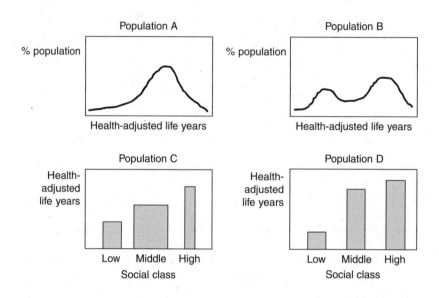

information instead of simply inequality information, I use the term 'health inequality measurement.' This is because I believe that the process of quantifying equity information asks distinct questions, which always emerge when we try to quantify any information worthy of assessment.[2]

A health inequality measurement summarizes a health distribution into one number and expresses the degree of health inequality. Summarizing the extent of inequality in a health distribution by means of a single number facilitates examination, comparison, and understanding of the health inequality in question. This summary process inevitably requires selection, suppression, and omission of certain information carried by a health distribution. The decision to select a specific aspect of health inequality may be influenced by such various factors as epidemiological and economic knowledge, policy relevance, and moral considerations (Kaplow 2002). Most questions that arise when summarizing a health distribution into one number are, as already mentioned, distinct. Whatever perspectives on health equity one might choose, measuring it requires addressing further questions. As we will see below, the perspectives discussed in the previous chapters rarely assist us in answering these questions.

A variety of health inequality measurements have been routinely used, including range measures, the Gini coefficient, and the World Health Organization (WHO) health inequality index. Each of these measurements summarizes a particular set of information that a health distribution carries. This means that even when it is used for the same health distribution, each measurement focuses on a different aspect of the health distribution. As a result, the degree of health inequality may differ depending on the measurement. Different results could lead to different policy implications. The decision to use a specific health inequality measure is too important to be made on the basis of convenience alone. To choose an appropriate health inequality measure properly, we must understand the summary process.

The purpose of this chapter is, therefore, to clarify the choices that must be made in summarizing a health distribution into one number. The plan of this chapter is as follows. I first discuss the importance of recognizing inequality as a complex notion and whether health inequality should be measured alone or with other population health goals. Second, building upon the relevant literature in economics, philosophy, and health sciences, I consider five questions that arise in summarizing a health distribution into one number. Through examining these five questions one by one, I identify properties that health inequality measures should satisfy. Finally, I make recommendations for selecting among various health inequality measurements.

As I warned in the introduction, this is the most demanding chapter in the book. The reason is that this chapter bridges philosophy and numbers and symbolizes the excitingly multidisciplinary nature of health inequality measurement. Therefore, non-quantitative readers may find the numbers difficult to follow, while quantitative readers may be puzzled by my philosophical analysis of the numbers. I try my best for clear explanation, but I also ask readers for patience. I suggest that those who wish to avoid detailed discussion skip the entire section 4.4.

4.2 Preliminaries

Inequality, a Complex Notion

We can assess health inequality objectively and normatively. Objectively, we say which inequality is less, while normatively, we judge which inequality is worse. Such thinkers as Sen are sceptical about the conceptual separability of the objective and normative notions of inequality (1997, 2–3). Their argument goes as follows: it is an objective, that is,

Figure 4.2 Disagreement between health inequality measures

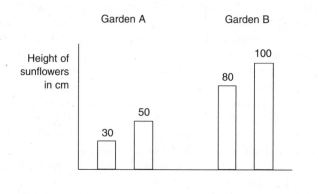

	Garden A	Garden B
Absolute difference	50 − 30 = 20	100 − 80 = 20
Relative difference	50 / 30 = 1.67	100 / 80 = 1.25

a factual description to say that a 50/50 division of a cake is an equal division or that two people both having lived 60 years are equal in terms of the length of life. When a situation becomes complex, however, it seems impossible to express inequality objectively. Imagine a six-person world, for example, each member of which lived 30, 30, 40, 40, 40, and 60 years, respectively. How equal is this population in terms of length of life? Imagine further another six-person world whose distribution of the length of life is 20, 20, 60, 60, 70, and 70 years. Which population is more equal in terms of the length of life, and by how much? Sen and others would argue that the statement that each of these populations is unequal in terms of the length of life is objective, but any further statements about the equality of situations like these inevitably go beyond objectivity and require value judgments.

Is this claim true? That is, are objective and normative notions inseparable in our thinking about inequality? I am dubious of this claim. For many distributions, we cannot easily answer which distribution is more equal, but the inability to answer does not mean that there is no answer. However complex they might be, I believe that there are both objective and normative notions of inequality. I think that the difficulties derive from the complexity of the objective notion of inequality.

It is widely known that different inequality measures can imply different degrees of inequality for the same distribution (Wagstaff, Paci, and van Doorslaer 1991). This is true even in a simple, descriptive case. Suppose there are two gardens, A and B, each consisting of two sunflowers. We are interested in the inequality of height between these flowers (see fig. 4.2). To express a degree of inequality in each garden, one might use simple inequality measures, such as the absolute difference and the relative difference.

These two simple inequality measures, despite their intention to merely describe inequality, suggest different degrees of inequality. Inequalities in the height of sunflowers in Garden A and B are the same if measured by the absolute difference (A: 50 – 30 = 20; B: 100 – 80 = 20), while Garden A presents more inequality than Garden B if measured by the relative difference (A: 50/30 = 1.67; B: 100/80 = 1.25). Though one might prefer one measure to the other based on aesthetic, technical, biological, or economic grounds, both are legitimate inequality measures. Such disagreement among inequality measures implies that the notion of inequality is complex (Temkin 1993).

An ideal inequality measure would be an objective measure that captures all aspects of the complex notion of inequality and tells us what is 'as a matter of empirical fact,' the 'true' degree of inequality (Oppenheim 1970). In the case of the sunflower example above, an ideal inequality measure would capture both our judgment that Garden A and B are equal in terms of the height of sunflowers (expressed in the absolute difference) as well as our judgment that they are not (expressed in the relative difference). The fact that we have not succeeded in identifying such an ideal measure, even in this simple case, suggests that there is a tremendous challenge in investigating the complex notion of inequality. Furthermore, disagreement between inequality measures regarding the degree of inequality indicates that each of them only captures some aspects of the complex notion of inequality. In other words, each of the inequality measures currently available is incomplete as an objective measure.

Is there any way to construct an objective inequality measure that captures all the aspects of complex inequality? There has, in fact, been such an attempt in income inequality measurement, the intersection approach, proposed by Sen (1997, 72–4). Very briefly, the intersection approach uses a number of inequality measures and ranks distributions only when different inequality measures agree with one another in their rankings. When inequality measures disagree, ranking is not assigned to a distribution, thus the approach is called 'quasi-ordering.' [3] This effort to reflect the complexity of the objective notion of inequality comes at considerable cost, as the intersection approach often cannot rank the inequalities of all the distributions in which we are interested, and, even when it does, all information we can obtain about inequality is ranking. Such a policy-relevant question as how much more (or less) inequality there is is beyond its reach.

In addition, the intersection approach might be especially difficult to apply to health inequality. The intersection approach was originally proposed for measuring income inequality. Health is presumably a more complex good than income. It is true that measurement of income has such complicated issues as sources and taxes, but the complexity of measurement of health may be much greater. Despite the lack of clear agreement over the number and nature of the dimensions health consists of, it is reasonable to assume that health is multidimensional. Depending on the health dimension selected, the degree of health inequality differs (Anand et al. 2001). We have no gold standard for the measurement of health, and the degree of health inequality is likely to change according to the different measurements of health used. By accounting for the multidimensionality of health, how many distributions does the intersection approach ultimately rank? Perhaps not many. As a strategy, the intersection approach is most likely to be implausible for measuring health inequality.[4]

What alternatives do we have? One strategy is to accept that we can focus on only certain aspects of health inequality and be explicit about the choice (Atkinson 1983, 56; Broome 1989; Dalton 1920). By deciding to focus on a particular aspect of inequality, we will not try to accommodate all aspects of the presumably complex notion of health inequality. Popular health inequality measures, such as the range measures, the Concentration Index, and the Gini coefficient, are only such partial measures (Wagstaff 2002a), but their users rarely pay attention to the information selected, suppressed, and omitted. Without understanding this summary process, which involves value judgment, one cannot assess which health inequality measure might be better suited to summarize a health distribution.

What to Measure – Inequality Alone or with the Population's Mean Health?

Some researchers contend that one should always deal with health inequality as an equity–efficiency trade-off (Williams and Cookson 2000). By doing so, they say, one avoids even contemplating the unacceptable option of realizing health equality by harming the healthy (Williams 1997b, 346).[5] They rightly argue that one should think about the costs of reducing health inequality in terms of the sacrifice of other goods. From this point of view, health inequality should be measured within a social welfare function, where one can incorporate social preference for health equality as compared to other ideals (often expressed by a parameter of inequality aversion; we will discuss this later in the discussion on aggregation) into a larger social welfare framework.[6]

In the actual policy-making process, it may indeed be better to examine health inequality simultaneously with other considerations. Yet even in this case, one must have a clear idea about health inequality itself. Selecting appropriate aspects of health inequality is in itself complex. The estimation of a social welfare function cannot avoid this complex process; it requires a clear understanding of health inequality before taking the additional task of assigning the relative value of equality among other ideals. Thus, in this chapter I focus on measuring health inequality alone instead of measuring it with such other considerations as the average health of the population.

What is interesting and puzzling, though, is the ambiguity surrounding the exact boundary of considerations of inequality. As we see below, for example, there has been an argument over whether income and health inequality measures should be sensitive to the mean in a given population.[7] There is, in other words, no agreement upon whether consideration of a population's mean level is within or outside the consideration of inequality. Temkin doubts the conceptual separability of our thinking on inequality and the mean (Temkin 1993, 202–6). As Sen says, a good measurement is a good reflection of our conception (1997, 5–6). If in our mind the mean and inequality are not completely separable, health inequality measurements should reflect such inseparability. In the following discussion, I accept the possibility that the extent of inequality depends on the mean.

4.3 The Five Questions: An Overview

I propose to consider the following five questions that arise when summarizing a health distribution into one number:

1 Comparison: who is compared against whom?
2 Aggregation: how are differences aggregated at the population level?

3 Sensitivity to the mean: should the judgment of inequality be sensitive to the mean level of the population?
4 Sensitivity to the population size: should the judgment of inequality
be sensitive to the total population size?
5 Subgroup considerations: should the judgment of inequality be sensitive to the subpopulation size, and how should the overall inequality of a population correspond to inequalities of subgroups in that
population?

Various considerations come into play when examining these questions, for example, policy relevance, epidemiological and economic
knowledge, and moral concerns. By answering them, we select certain
information carried by a health distribution. Answers to these questions, in other words, form the backbone of health inequality measurement.

I do not include the unit of analysis in the list above, although it is
clearly an important consideration when selecting a health inequality
measure. I discussed it in chapter 3 because of its strong connection
to the question of how we characterize health in the pursuit of its
equalization. These five key questions are relevant whichever unit of
analysis – individual or group – one might select.

Indeed, these five questions are appropriate irrespective of the choice
of a health measurement and unit of time. In this chapter, I assume
Health-adjusted Life Years (HALYs) as the health about whose distribution we are concerned. HALYs combine life years and quality of life.
This reflects the conclusion in chapter 3 that functionality and general
symptoms should be the focus of health in health equity analysis
(quality of life in HALYs is measured by health status measures, which
also focus on functionality and general symptoms). But for the purpose
of this chapter, my choice of health measurement could be anything;
whatever measurement of health is selected, these five questions would
always arise, and we would examine them as this chapter does. Similarly,
although I use the whole-life approach for its simplicity, discussions in
this chapter apply to any choice of the unit of time.

A perceptive reader might still be suspicious over whether these five
questions always arise in any perspectives on health equity. For example,
are these questions still valid when one is interested in measuring
health inequality according to the view of equity as satisfying the minimally adequate level of health? Poverty measures, which have a close
affiliation to this equity perspective, often do not only count how many

people are below the threshold but also consider the distribution below it (Sen 1997, 164–94). If one acknowledges the merit of this procedure, it does not take long to recognize that these five questions do arise below the threshold (see appendix E2 for further elaboration).

Just by looking at the questions, it should be clear that most of them are different kinds of questions than the ones we examined in the previous chapters. This means that the choice of perspective on health equity would not always guide us in answering these questions. Most of these questions are distinct. Nonetheless, whenever possible, I try to clarify possible connections we could make between these questions and different equity perspectives.

I am not the first to isolate these questions. The so-called axiomatic approach in the income inequality literature has examined various axioms, which can be considered particular answers to some of the five questions above. Specifically in the health context, researchers have also discussed these five questions singly or in combination with varying emphases.[8] In addition, although not paying particular attention to health, Temkin discusses them from a philosophical perspective (1993). My contribution here is to identify the most appropriate questions for the measurement of health inequality and attempt to find the best answer to each question. Difficulty in answering these questions often leads to the recommendation to use various inequality measures in analysis (for example, Williams and Doessel 2006). Sensitivity analysis has a merit, of course, and pluralism at a time of uncertainty is sensible. But I expect that there might be some answers we can reasonably support.

How can we then examine these five questions? We can investigate them empirically and philosophically. The empirical investigation often employs questionnaires asking how a sample of people thinks about inequalities by presenting various hypothetical distributional scenarios. The philosophical investigation explores and examines our intuitive feelings about different distributions. Why do we think in this particular way and what should we think?

In the income inequality measurement research, the empirical approach plays a unique role in discovering that people do not often agree with standard distributional axioms upon which many income inequality measures are built.[9] The empirical approach is also emerging in health sciences research. This is not surprising given that the empirical approach is so popular in constructing a health status measure. In constructing the WHO health inequality index, for example, Gakidou,

Murray, and Frenk conducted a computer-based questionnaire consisting of twenty-nine questions with verbal and graphical presentations of health distributions, and constructed its health inequality measure based on the survey results from 1007 respondents, within which 501 were the WHO staff (Gakidou, Murray, and Frenk 2001). Health inequality measures and health status measures present many similar issues of value elicitation, for example, who we should ask – the general public, experts, or the sick – and in what way – by mail, telephone, or Internet. In addition, graphical representation of questions is no doubt challenging.[10]

I believe both empirical and philosophical approaches are necessary for investigating the aforementioned five questions. On the one hand, knowing what people think is a good starting point to investigate why they think so. If we believe inequality measurements should reflect ideas shared in society, it is alarming that standard distributional axioms do not reflect what people think. It is hard to justify their predominant use. Although this finding is from surveys on income inequality, we can expect that the same might be true for health inequality.

On the other hand, 'empirical ethics' – what the majority of people think about – should not be the sole guide of our morality (Hausman 2002). Some questions are difficult, and our true ideas may not be revealed by opinion surveys. If our notion of inequality was indeed complex, questions regarding health inequality would be very demanding. More importantly, even if a survey could collect opinions of what people really think, the majority opinion would not always be the best social choice we should make. Furthermore, philosophical investigation could provide at least an initial framework with which we could construct a questionnaire and investigate survey responses.

My approach in this project is primarily philosophical. But whenever it is informative, I touch on the empirical investigations of others, especially the WHO's health inequality questionnaire.

Throughout this chapter, I use five popular health inequality measures as examples. These five health inequality measures are, as summarized in table 4.1, the range measures, the Concentration Index, the generalized Concentration Index, the Gini coefficient, and the WHO health inequality index. I chose these five health inequality measures for a variety of reasons. The range measures are the simplest health inequality measure and, thus, a good start to examine the five questions arising in the process of summarizing a distribution into one number. Despite the criticism of being too crude (Sen 1997, 25; Wagstaff, Paci, and van Doorslaer 1991), they are still commonly used. The Concentration Index is recommended by Wagstaff, Paci, and van Doorslaer (1991) as preferable measures of health inequality across socio-economic status and has gained popularity.[11] The generalized Concentration Index is a close cousin of the Concentration Index. Illsley and Le Grand are pioneers in measuring health inequality across individuals, and the Gini coefficient was one of their choices of inequality measurements in their early studies (Illsley and Le Grand 1987; Le Grand 1987). The WHO health inequality index is controversial in various aspects but has provoked a number of stimulating discussions.[12] See appendix A for a detailed explanation of these five inequality measures. By focusing only on the five inequality measures, this chapter does not provide readers with an exhaustive list of health inequality measures. Yet I believe these five inequality measures serve as sufficient examples to show core issues in selecting or creating a health inequality measure among numerous inequality measures available.[13]

4.4 The Five Questions: A Close Look

Now we look at the five questions one by one. To help connect the conceptual discussion with its numerical expression, at the beginning of each question I list the Gini coefficient as an example of a health inequality measure and highlight a mathematical expression relevant to each question. Although the relationships between these five questions are likely to be important, I discuss each question separately unless otherwise stated.

Comparison

How many units should one compare, and who is compared against whom in the population?

$$G = \frac{1}{2} \sum_{i=1}^{n} \sum_{j=1}^{n} \frac{|y_i - y_j|}{n^2 \mu}$$

G: the Gini coefficient, where the population of interest holds n people, y_i is the health of individual i, y_j is the health of individual j, and the average level of health in the population is μ.

How many units should one compare, and who is compared against whom in the population? Anand and his colleagues refer to the group

Table 4.1
Selected health inequality measures

	Expression	Interpretation	Examples
Number of units = 2			
Range measures			
Ratio	$R = \dfrac{\mu_1}{\mu_2}$	The average health of group 1 is X times higher/lower than that of group 2	Low and Low (2006), Machenbach and Kunst (1997)
Absolute difference	$A = \mu_1 - \mu_2$	The average health of group 1 is X-unit more/less than that of group 2	Low and Low (2006), Machenbach and Kunst (1997)
Shortfalls in Achievement	$SFA = \dfrac{\mu_g - Y_{min}}{Y_{max} - Y_{min}}$	The average health of group g is X times higher/lower than the norm	Anand and Sen (1994, 1995), Norheim (2006)
Number of units > 2, measures of health inequality in relation to other characteristic (for example, socio-economic status)			
The Concentration Index	$C = \dfrac{2}{n\mu} \sum_{i=1}^{n} y_i R_i - 1$	C (or GC) = −1: the population's entire health is concentrated in people in the socially most disadvantaged group C (or GC) = 0: perfect equality	van Doorslaer and Koolman (2004), Humphries and van Doorslaer (2000)
The generalized Concentration Index	$GC = \dfrac{2}{n} \sum_{i=1}^{n} y_i R_i - 1$	C (or GC) = 1: the population's entire health is concentrated in people in the socially most advantaged group	

Table 4.1 (continued)

	Expression	Interpretation	Examples
Number of units >2, measures of health inequality across individuals			
The Gini coefficient	$G = \dfrac{1}{2} \sum_{i=1}^{n} \sum_{j=1}^{n} \dfrac{\lvert y_i - y_j \rvert}{n^2 \mu}$	$G = 0$: perfect equality $G = 1$: most unequal	Le Grand (1987) Illsley and Le Grand (1987)
The WHO health inequality index	$W = 1 - \sum_{i=1}^{n} \sum_{j=1}^{n} \dfrac{\lvert y_i - y_j \rvert^3}{2n^2 \mu^{0.5}}$	$W = 0$: worst inequality that has ever been measured in any country $W = 1$: perfect equality	World Health Organization (2000)

Y_{max}: the maximum health or the health norm
Y_{min}: the minimum health possible
μ: the average health of the entire population
$\mu_g (g = 1,2)$: the average health of the group g
$R_i (i = 1,....,n)$: the relative rank of the ith person (individuals are ranked from the most disadvantaged socio-economically to the advantaged)
n: the number of people in the entire population
$y_i (i = 1,....,n)$: health of the ith person
$y_j (j = 1,....,n)$: health of the jth person

Figure 4.3   Comparison concepts

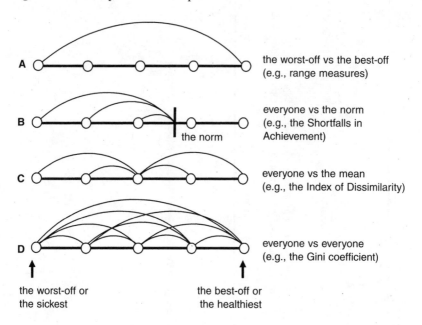

A   the worst-off vs the best-off
(e.g., range measures)

B   everyone vs the norm
(e.g., the Shortfalls in
Achievement)
the norm

C   everyone vs the mean
(e.g., the Index of Dissimilarity)

D   everyone vs everyone
(e.g., the Gini coefficient)

the worst-off or   the best-off or
the sickest   the healthiest

or person compared against as a 'reference' (2001). A simple illustration might help clarify this first question. Suppose we are interested in
health inequality within a population consisting of five people. Let us
line them up horizontally from the sickest to the healthiest or the worst-
off to the best-off. In figure 4.3 a small circle represents a person or a
group, and arcs between them represent the comparisons one makes.
Next to the illustration, figure 4.3 also provides examples of popular
health inequality measures that apply to each of the comparison concepts. Obviously, numerous comparison concepts exist, and more may
be created. These four choices are not exhaustive and are intended only
to illustrate the discussion points.

Which comparison concept might be appropriate for health inequality measures? Range measures that use the comparison concept A are
often criticized as rough measures of inequality (Sen 1997, 25; Wagstaff,
Paci, and van Doorslaer 1991). But the simplicity of comparing only two
groups, the worst-off and the best-off or the sickest and the healthiest,
can produce a straightforward, strong message, and range measures

would be the best comparison concept for the purpose of sending out an urgent message of health inequality. In addition, when one is interested in the health of a specific person or group, it is natural to focus on them in one's measurements. The health of the poor, for example, has traditionally been an important policy focus (Gwatkin, Guillot, and Heuveline 1999; Gwatkin and Heuveline 1999; Wagstaff 2002b), and it is reasonable to presume that those who have a special interest in the health of the poor would wish their health inequality measure to reflect it.

Comparison concept B is typically applied to a comparison of two units, that is, one group or individual against a norm representing a policy objective or reflecting what is achievable (Anand and Sen 1994; Anand and Sen 1995; Sen 1992, chap. 6). An optimal health achievement is often set as a norm, for example, the lowest infant mortality rate observed in the world, to see how far off the norm is the infant mortality rate of the population of interest. This comparison concept can also be used for more than two comparison units; one can compare anyone below the norm against the norm (Norheim 2006). Comparison concept B might thus be attractive to those who believe a right to basic health exists. There is an obvious similarity between poverty measures and health inequality measures using the comparison concept B. If one were interested in developing this path, poverty measures would provide good guidance.

As illustrated in comparison concept C, the mean level of health of a population is sometimes selected as the norm against which the comparison is made (Mackenbach 1993; Pappas et al. 1993). Why should the mean be set as a norm? In the case of income and welfare, one might think that a society produces a certain amount of wealth, and the fair share is an equal share. Thus, the average level can be a norm (Temkin 1993, 20). Though health is only partially redistributable, one might make the analogy to health. As Anand and his colleagues pointed out (2001, 53), however, it is puzzling that health above the mean diminishes equality to just the same extent as health below the mean.

Comparison concept D acknowledges any differences in health observed in a population. This thoroughness is the attraction of choice D, and there are two rather different reasons to favour it. The first is related to our idea of the degree of thoroughness a good inequality measure should have. If one wanted to measure the inequality between the height of sunflowers in a garden thoroughly, one would count them all. The same would apply to measure inequality in the health of humans. If one does not have a special interest in a particular person or group or a specific norm in mind, almost as a default, it would be best to compare everyone's health.

In this view, comparison concept D might appear to be the most objective choice. But this appearance is deceiving; often this choice implies a moral position. The second reason to approve this concept's thoroughness is moral.

In his painstaking analysis of when one situation is worse than another in terms of inequality, Temkin proposed to view a distribution from the perspective of individuals (1993). In a population that exhibits an unequal distribution, someone is unsatisfied with her share relative to others' and has a 'complaint.'[14] A complaint about a low level of health may not help us think any further, but consider what the lack of health could mean to the person. She lacks an important resource that will be effective for whatever life plan she may have, and her welfare level itself is likely to be low. Because ill health could be compensated for with other resources or welfare components, her unsatisfactory health is not inevitably burdensome. Still, in this case too she can have a complaint at the need for compensating resources, while others with better health need not be bothered. Counting any differences in health observed in a population is to acknowledge any complaints brought by anyone in the population. These two perspectives make a strong case in support of comparison concept D when there is no special interest in the health of a particular person or group.

Which comparison concept, then, should a health inequality measure use? Unless one has a particular interest in a specific person or group (for example, the worst-off) or a certain norm (for example, the minimally adequate level of health), concept D would be most appropriate for health inequality measures: everyone's health should be compared against everyone's health.[15]

Aggregation

How are differences aggregated at the population level?

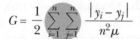

$$G = \frac{1}{2} \sum_{i=1}^{n} \sum_{j=1}^{n} \frac{|y_i - y_j|}{n^2 \mu}$$

When deciding who is compared against whom in a population, one identifies the difference(s) on which each health inequality measure focuses. When one compares more than two units, a question arises

Figure 4.4   Aggregation of differences

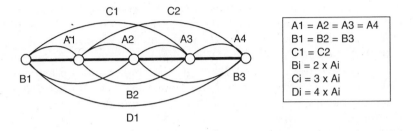

concerning how each difference is aggregated at the population level. This is related to the question about how we 'value health differently along the distribution' (Anand et al. 2001, 54–5). Suppose once again a population consisting of five people whose HALYs are equally distanced. If we use the comparison concept D above, in which everyone's health is compared against everyone's health, we need somehow to combine A1, A2, A3, A4, B1, B2, B3, C1, C2, and D1 in figure 4.4.

To obtain the total difference in a population, there are a large number of ways to aggregate all differences. The most common method of aggregation is addition, and one must make a choice between unweighted and weighted addition. In unweighted addition of differences one adds all differences as they are, while in weighted addition of differences one adds them with some sort of weighting attached. Most popular health inequality measures, including the Concentration Index and the Gini coefficient, use unweighted addition of differences. The WHO health inequality index is an exception: it adds each difference cubed. In developing the WHO health inequality index, Gakidou, Murray, and Frenk introduced a parameter α – each difference is raised to the power of α – to respond to the question of the 'intensity of health gain/loss' (Gakidou, Murray, and Frenk 2000). When $\alpha = 1$, all differences are unweighted. The greater the value of α is, the more accentuated larger differences are. Reflecting results of a survey, they set $\alpha = 3$ (Gakidou, Murray, and Frenk 2001).[16]

The above explanation concerns weighting *differences*. Alternatively, one can think of how much weight should be attached to each person's (or group's) *share of health*. One can interpret, for example, the Concentration Index and the Gini coefficient as attaching weight to each

person's (or group's) health share according to his or her rank and
summing the rank-order-weighted health shares. In this interpretation,
it turns out that these two measures give decreasing weights from
the lowest to the highest ranked person (or group), and the weight
attached to the lowest rank is two and the highest rank zero (Wagstaff
2002a). Some scholars think that this weighting scheme is arbitrary and
have suggested the extended Concentration Index and the extended
Gini coefficient (Bleichrodt and van Doorslaer 2006; Norheim 2006;
Wagstaff 2002a; Yitzhaki 1983), which can incorporate different weighting schemes into the measurement as users wish. To reflect 'distributional sensitivity' (Bleichrodt and van Doorslaer 2006, 947), these
extended measures have introduced the parameter v. When $v=1$, each
health share is equally weighted, and however unequal a distribution is,
these extended inequality measures judge that the distribution is perfectly equal. When the parameter v takes values greater than 1, these
extended inequality measures reflect greater concerns towards the
lower end of the distribution.[17] The priority view (Parfit 1991), briefly
introduced in section 2.2 of chapter 2, can be expressed with such
weighting.

Despite the different framing as described above, the heart of the
aggregation issue is whether we wish to value distances along the distribution differently, depending on the location and size of differences.
The issue of location, for example, is whether A1 should be treated as
identical to A4 in figure 4.4. Or should we treat the health share of each
of the five people in the same way? The question of size is, similarly,
whether C1 should be treated as exactly three times larger than A1.

I believe our moral concern for health distribution suggests some
asymmetric weighting in terms of location but not the size of differences. Temkin's view of understanding each difference as a complaint
provides a hint (1993, chap. 2). Each of the five individuals in figure
4.4 has complaints against all those who are healthier than herself. If
expressed in the absolute difference of HALYs, the complaint that the
sickest has against the second sickest is the same as the second healthiest has against the healthiest. But one might want to place different
weights on the same HALYs or where a person stands along the distribution, depending on whether they are at the lower or higher tails
of the distribution. On the other hand, a longer distance already
suggests a larger complaint, and it is unclear why we might wish to at-
tach an additional weight to a larger complaint. Is it not enough to

acknowledge the difference in health between people as the distance itself indicates?[18]

Both the parameters α (introduced for the WHO health inequality index by Gakidou, Murray, and Frenk [2001]) and v (introduced for the extended Concentration Index and Gini coefficient by Wagstaff [2002a] and Bleichrodt and van Doorslaer [2006]) can express asymmetric weighting. Despite the difference between weighting differences (α) and weighting health shares (v), inequality measures using these parameters behave similarly at least in some parameter values (Norheim 2006),[19] for example, both $\alpha = 1$ and $v = 2$ give the standard Concentration Index and Gini coefficient. Values $v = 2$ and $\alpha = 1$ suggest, respectively, that the standard Concentration Index and Gini coefficient provide asymmetric weighting in terms of location but do not weight differences. Thus, the standard Concentration Index and Gini coefficient happen to express what our moral concern for health distribution suggests.

Should one wish to express even greater concern towards the lower ends of the distribution and even some concern for larger differences, one could adopt either a greater value for v in the extended Concentration Index and Gini coefficient or a value for greater than 1 as the WHO health inequality index does. An important question is exactly what kind of asymmetric weighting we wish to adopt, or what should be the value of v or α.

In introducing such a parameter as v, economists often argue that users of inequality measurement should be able to reflect their own normative position in the measurement. While I agree with the importance of the consistency from the normative position to measurement, I worry about giving options to change a parameter without clarifying what such a number really means. Our moral concern for health distribution appears to suggest some sort of asymmetric weighting, but presently we do not know how exactly such asymmetric weighting should take shape. We need to further explore Temkin's proposal to understand the difference as a complaint in the health inequality context and how best it is expressed in health inequality measurement. In addition, we need to investigate further how our moral concerns for differences and health share might relate to each other. Moreover, the issue of aggregation eventually needs to be addressed with other issues, for example, the sensitivity to the mean, or even how weighting in health inequality measurement might relate to weighting in measurement of health.

Sensitivity to the Mean[20]

Should the judgment of inequality be sensitive to the mean level of the population?

$$G = \frac{1}{2} \sum_{i=1}^{n} \sum_{j=1}^{n} \frac{|y_i - y_j|}{n^2 \mu}$$

Sensitivity to the mean is an interesting issue for its suggestion that it is not always easy to separate inequality judgments from such other ideals as maximization of the average. The question of sensitivity to the mean has been discussed as one of the key questions that emerge in the process of summarizing a distribution.[21] Despite this widespread discussion, the results are often confusing. I believe that further clarification is necessary, especially in the health context. The discussion in this section assumes the use of a positive health measure, by which a population with a higher mean level of health is a healthier population.

THE SAME MEAN, DIFFERENT DISTRIBUTIONS

At the risk of stating the obvious, many different distributions have the same mean. We must start with this recognition when investigating sensitivity to the mean of inequality measures.

Two types of the mean difference are often discussed: the equal proportional difference and the equal absolute difference. Figure 4.5 illustrates them with examples of simple two-person populations.[22] Both people in Population B have 25 HALYs more and both people in Population D have 50 HALYs more than the people in Population A. Thus, Population A and B, and A and D have equal absolute differences. The HALYs of both people in Population C are twice those of the members of A, and those of the people in Population E are three times those of the people in Population A. Population A and C, and A and E, therefore, have equal proportional differences. Notice that Population B and C, and D and E have the same means though their distributions are different. This simple point, as we will see below, is important in thinking of the issue of sensitivity to the mean. In the discussion of sensitivity to the mean, one must always ask: in what way is the mean different between populations?

TWO TYPES OF THE MEAN DIFFERENCE AND THREE RESPONSES
FROM INEQUALITY MEASURES

Corresponding to these two types of the mean difference, inequality measures commonly respond to them in one of the following three ways:

Figure 4.5   Two types of the mean difference

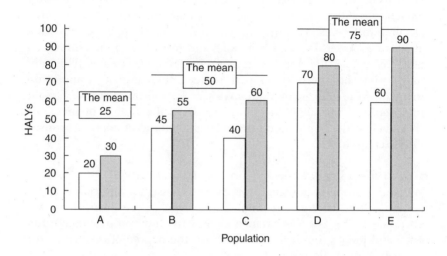

- Response 1: Equal proportional difference implies equal degree of inequality ($I_A=I_C=I_E$ in figure 4.5), while the equal absolute addition reduces inequality ($I_A>I_B>I_D$).
- Response 2: Equal absolute difference implies equal degree of inequality ($I_A=I_B=I_D$), while the equal proportional increase makes inequality larger ($I_A<I_C<I_E$).
- Response 3: Equal proportional increase makes inequality bigger ($I_A<I_C<I_E$), while equal absolute addition decreases inequality ($I_A>I_B>I_D$).

The property of insensitivity to the equal proportional difference of Response 1 is called the scale invariance. This is one type of mean-independence. Inequality measures with this property are often referred to as relative or intensive measures. This property is attractive to those who measure income inequality, because it implies that the degree of inequality does not change due to inflation or different monetary units. The property of insensitivity to equal absolute difference of Response 2 is called the translation invariance. This is the other type of mean-independence. Inequality measures with this property are referred to as absolute or equal-invariant measures.

Response 3 was first proposed by Dalton as early as in 1920. He calls

it the Principle of Equal Additions to Incomes (1920). Kolm metaphor-
ically terms measures that are insensitive to equal proportional difference as 'rightist' measures and ones that are insensitive to equal
absolute difference as 'leftist' measures (1976). He proposes the same
alternative view as Dalton's principle, and he calls such measures 'cen-
trist,' regarding their location as between the two extremes. This alternative view has been developed under the name of 'compromise
inequality' or 'intermediate inequality.'[23] Furthermore, Temkin, in his
philosophical investigation of how sensitive the notion of inequality
should be to the population's mean level, seems to endorse Response 3
(1993, chap. 6).

MEAN-INDEPENDENCE — WHAT DOES IT REALLY MEAN?

When the property of scale invariance or translation invariance is concerned, often the focus is only on one type of the mean difference
(Broome 1989). Scale invariance deals with equal proportional difference and judges that it has no effect on the degree of inequality. It is
often forgotten, however, that inequality measures with this property
also make another judgment: that equal absolute addition reduces
inequality. Similarly, translation invariance looks at the equal absolute
difference and judges that it has no effect on the degree of inequality.
But attention is rarely paid to the fact that measures with this property
also judge that equal proportional increase makes inequality bigger. An
inequality measure cannot simultaneously and perfectly satisfy both
types of mean-independence. In other words, if an inequality measure
is mean-independent in terms of equal proportional difference, it is not
mean-independent in terms of equal absolute difference, and vice
versa. This point can be easily shown by simple examples.

Table 4.2 summarizes degrees of inequality of the two-person
populations A, B, C, D, and E in figure 4.5 measured both by absolute
difference and relative difference measures. Absolute differences are
measured in units. For example, in Population A there is a 10-HALY
absolute difference between the two persons. Relative differences, on
the other hand, express their quantities proportionally and not in units.
For example, in Population A one person's HALYs are 1.5 times longer
than the other. Both are relational in a sense that calculation is only possible when one is compared against another.

The absolute difference measure judges that inequalities in Population A, B, and D are the same, obviously because they have the equal
absolute difference between them. But according to this measure this is

Table 4.2
Disagreement between health inequality measures

Population	A	B	C	D	E
Mean	25	50	50	75	75
Absolute difference	10	10	20	10	30
Relative difference	1.5	1.2	1.5	1.1	1.5

Inequality judgment
   Absolute difference measure: $I_A = I_B = I_D$, $I_A < I_C < I_E$
   Relative difference measure: $I_A = I_C = I_E$, $I_D < I_B < I_A$

not the case for Population C and E. Population C's inequality is greater than A's, and E's inequality is greater than C's. Similarly, the relative difference measure judges that inequalities in Population A, C, and E are the same given that they have the equal proportional difference, but not B and D. B's inequality is greater than D's, and A's inequality is greater than D's. The sensitivity to the mean in these two measures does not simply depend on the mean level but in what way the means are different.

Moreover, this simple example shows that the question of sensitivity to the mean is not merely whether an inequality measure has a mean term in its formula but how it perceives differences in health.[24] In thinking of how much health inequality exists in Population A, for example, if one looks at the difference, 20 HALYs and 30 HALYs, relatively, one is already making an assumption that equal proportional difference has no impact on inequality while the equal absolute addition reduces inequality (Response 1 above). On the other hand, if one perceives the difference absolutely, one is making an assumption that equal absolute difference does not change the degree of inequality but equal proportional increase makes inequality bigger (Response 2 above). Similarly, if one perceives the difference in some mix of the absolute and relative difference, one is making an assumption that equal proportional increase makes inequality bigger while equal absolute addition decreases inequality (Response 3 above). Perceiving a difference between people by absolute or relative difference embeds a certain sensitivity to the mean level. The question we must answer is not whether we wish our inequality measure to be sensitive to the population's mean level but in what way we want it to be sensitive.

The term 'mean-independence' is commonly employed in the inequality measurement literature, but its usage is confusing. It is often

used as if there were only one way to be mean-independent, while there
are in fact at least two ways for an inequality measure to be mean-
independent (Temkin 1993, 181–2). In economics, insensitivity to equal
absolute difference is considered to be a more demanding property
than insensitivity to equal proportional difference, and many inequality
measures are constructed to satisfy this latter, less demanding, insensitivity. Consequently, inequality measures insensitive to equal proportional difference are customarily referred to as mean-independent
measures, which give the mistaken impression that they are insensitive
both to equal proportional difference and equal absolute difference.

HOW SHOULD HEALTH INEQUALITY MEASURES RESPOND TO
THE EQUAL PROPORTIONAL DIFFERENCE?

We have looked at three ways in which inequality measures respond to
two types of mean difference. Which of these three types of sensitivity to
the mean might be reasonable for a health inequality measure? Let us
first focus on equal proportional differences. Should equal proportional difference have any effect on the degree of health inequality?

I argue that equal proportional difference (Population A, C, and E in
figure 4.5) is not the kind of mean difference we should be worried
about in the assessment of health inequality. As discussed, it is understandable why researchers of the measurement of income inequality are
concerned about equal proportional difference. The concern is related
to the characteristics of the commodity on which they focus, money.
Equal proportional difference may, however, be less important for
health than income. Health does not have an inflation issue, for
example. Only when we measure health in different scales must we be
worried about equal proportional difference. We do not want, for
example, inequality in life expectancy to be different when measured in
life years or life months. As pointed out in the income inequality measurement context (Kakwani 1980, 65), this scale problem does not need
to be dealt with within inequality measurements; we can simply use the
same unit or adjust units for comparisons.

Putting the issue of health measurement scale aside, it is unlikely that
a health distribution changes equiproportionally (Le Grand 1987). And
comparing Population A, C, and E in figure 4.5, with the knowledge
that the same health measure is used for these populations, most would
agree that the equal proportional increase increases inequality. Applying Temkin's claim (1993, 181) to Population A, C, and E, if we
accepted that the allocation of the HALYs in Population A is problem-

atic, we would judge inequality in Population C to be bigger than in Population A as Population C is repeating the problematic allocation rule twice, and inequality in Population D is even bigger as it repeats it three times. Our assessment of health inequality seems to be sensitive to equal proportional difference, although further research is necessary to investigate exactly how sensitive it is. This suggests that scale invariance is not an appropriate property for health inequality measures, and thus, we reject Response 1 above.

HOW SHOULD HEALTH INEQUALITY MEASURES RESPOND TO THE
EQUAL ABSOLUTE DIFFERENCE?

Contrary to the equal proportional difference, the equal absolute difference seems to be closer to the mean difference we observe in health distributions. In addition, for the assessment of health inequality, perceiving a difference absolutely rather than relatively may provide useful information. Borrowing from epidemiology, absolute difference can be understood as attributable risk and relative differences as relative risk (Gordis 1996, 160–1; Mustard and Etches 2003). Attributable risk asks how much of a risk or a negative health outcome is attributable to a specific factor, and consequently, how much of a risk could be prevented if a specific factor was eliminated. Attributable risk, therefore, is useful for public and population health studies and clinical practice. Relative risk, on the other hand, asks whether there is any relationship between a risk and a specific factor, and if so, how strong it is. Relative risk, thus, is more suitable for etiological studies. In measuring health inequality, our interest is not etiological. We are instead interested in developing a tool that can help determine how great an impact an intervention can have on health inequality.[25]

To state the conclusion first, there seem to be good reasons to believe that our judgment of inequality is sensitive to equal absolute differences, that is, we may reasonably judge that the inequalities in Population A, B, and D are different and reject the property of the translation invariance. It is, however, unclear whether in our judgment equal absolute addition decreases or increases inequality and by how much.[26] To introduce different perspectives to make such arguments, for simplicity, I compare only Population A and D.

Kolm pays attention to the biological upper limit of human life. We do not know exactly what number of life years that is, but human life certainly is likely to have an upper limit, and Kolm points out that 'sufficient general progress in health mechanically tends to reduce inequality' (Kolm n.d., 21). This view suggests that it is easier to reduce health inequality at a higher mean, and we might wish to discount this biological effect. Given that the distributions of Population A and D in figure 4.5 are different only in terms of the mean levels, with the higher mean approaching an upper limit of human life, Population D could have done better than Population A. We might then want our health inequality measures to judge that Population D's inequality is greater than that of Population A. Note that Kolm's argument only applies to a very high mean, a population that challenges the biological upper limit.

Extending Kolm's biological explanation, the sentiment is often expressed that a healthier population (D) must have more resources than a less healthy population (A) and, using these resources, it must be easier for a healthier population to reduce inequality. According to this view, Population D should be penalized for the lack of effort to reduce inequality, and health inequality measures should judge Population D's inequality as greater than Population A's. Although this view might appear to be intuitively appealing, I doubt its validity. Empirical observations have shown little correlation between the mean and the degree of inequality in population health (World Health Organization 2000a). This casts doubt on the assumption that it must be easier to reduce inequality if more resources are available. Without this assumption, there is no reason to penalize Population D, and (unlike Kolm's account) this view does not offer any further explanation for why it might be easier for Population D to reduce inequality than Population A.

While Kolm brings a biological perspective, Temkin proposes a moral view. In his investigation of whether our notion of inequality should be sensitive to the overall population's level of affluence, he argues that the absolute difference between people does not of itself provide enough information because the same absolute difference is likely to have a greater impact on inequality in a less affluent society than in an affluent society (Temkin 1993, chap. 6). Applying Temkin's view to the health context, one might argue that the same absolute difference in health may mean more in a generally sicker population. That is, the difference of 10 HALYs in the population mean of 25 HALYs would weigh more than the same difference of 10 HALYs in the population mean of 75 HALYs. In short, Temkin's view suggests that given equal absolute differences, health inequality is greater in sicker populations.

It is interesting to see how different perspectives lead to different judgments in terms of the degree of inequality with equal absolute difference. This might suggest that our judgment on health inequality with equal absolute difference is not linear. We might think that inequality generally declines with equal absolute addition, yet at the very high mean level our judgment runs to the opposite. Unfortunately, we do not yet have a readily available means to reflect this view in health inequality measurement. But since Kolm's view only applies to a very high mean level, we may reasonably conclude that equal absolute addition in general decreases inequality.

INTERMEDIATE INEQUALITY AND HEALTH INEQUALITY MEASUREMENT

The preceding discussion suggests the following two points:

- Equal proportional increase increases health inequality.
- Equal absolute addition in general reduces health inequality.

Consequently, for the assessment of health inequality, the intermediate inequality notion, Response 3 above, is a reasonable choice.

The intermediate inequality concept is rarely employed in inequality measures used for the assessment of health inequality. The WHO health inequality index is a notable exception, and, interestingly, Gakidou, Murray, and Frenk opted for the intermediate inequality concept based on survey respondents' perceptions about sensitivity to the mean level. Although their pioneer role in empirically identifying the importance of the intermediate inequality concept deserves attention, much further work is necessary as to how the intermediate inequality concept can be appropriately expressed in a mathematical formulation of health inequality measurement. For example, to apply the intermediate inequality concept to health inequality measurement, one needs to identify *by how much* people think that the equal proportional increase makes health inequality bigger and *by how much* people think that the equal absolute addition reduces health inequality (see appendix B for a detailed explanation of how the WHO inequality index responds to these questions). These are not easy questions to explore, and both philosophical and empirical investigations are necessary.

Sensitivity to the Population Size

Should the judgment of inequality be sensitive to the total population size?

$$G = \frac{1}{2} \sum_{i=1}^{n} \sum_{j=1}^{n} \frac{|y_i - y_j|}{n^2 \mu}$$

Should the assessment of health inequality be sensitive to population size? Note that the focus here is not the proportional size of each group when using a group as the unit of analysis, but the size of the entire population in which either individuals or groups present a health distribution. Consider two populations with certain degrees of inequality that are then united. What is the degree of inequality of this total population? Putting this question into a context, suppose one has measures of health inequality in Canada and the United States. What then will be the degree of health inequality in the combination of the two? I suspect that interesting issues might arise in exploring this question, especially in the health context.[27] Along with the question of comparison, this question has some connection to questions we dealt with in the examination of perspectives on health equity.

It is generally believed that inequality of the total population is at least as great as or worse than inequality of any subpopulation (Kolm 1976, 100).[28] The reason is simple: we think of total inequality as consisting of inequality within a subpopulation and inequality between subpopulations. Thus, even if each of the two subpopulations had perfect equality, combining them would not always lead to perfect equality in the total population. Only if perfect equality in the two populations occurred at the same level would the total population be perfectly equal. Extended, the union of populations with the same distributional pattern and the mean, that is, replication, is generally considered to have no effect on the degree of inequality. This property is known as the Population Principle (Dalton 1920), and a large majority of inequality measures satisfy it.

Inequality measures that satisfy this Population Principle allow interpretation in per capita terms. This interpretation is obvious from formulae that include the population term, more precisely, the number of comparison units compared within the population (n) in the denominator. If we adopted Temkin's understanding of a complaint, for example, we could interpret inequality measured in this way as an average amount of complaint per person within a population. Alternatively, the population squared in the denominator (n^2) of the Gini coefficient or the WHO health inequality index formulae suggests that we can interpret inequality as results of random drawings with replacements (Foster 1985): we randomly choose two people from the population, keep a record of their difference in health, and put them back into the population.

This is certainly an attractive feature of the Population Principle, and perhaps for this reason the principle has rarely been questioned. Temkin, nonetheless, doubts that this principle deserves the universal application it currently enjoys (1993, chap. 7). He argues that the desirability of the Population Principle is determined by the reason for our primary interest in inequality. When the reason for our interest in inequality is social justice, our focus should be the pattern of inequality, not its size, thereby the Population Principle is acceptable (1993, 193–4). If, on the other hand, our concern for social justice is not the primary reason for investigating inequality, the Population Principle should be rejected. The reason, according to Temkin, is that even when two populations maintain the same pattern of inequalities, one population having more people suffering might bother us more, and this might influence our conception of inequality (1993, 200–2).

Temkin's view is worth considering in the health inequality context because sickness and suffering are often correlated. Thinking of the desirability of the Population Principle in health inequality measurement draws us back to a fundamental question: why are we interested in measuring health inequality? Social justice could be the primary reason for many people, but social justice does not need to be the sole reason why we are interested in health inequality. Lack of health could be associated with suffering, and, if so, one might consider that health inequality is greater in a larger population.

A crucial problem with this view is a bizarre conclusion it brings (Temkin 1993, 218–27; Williams and Cookson 2000). Imagine a comparison between a small population with a huge difference in health between people and a gigantic population with a trivial difference in health between people. Although differences in terms of health among members of the gigantic population may not be much, the suffering associated with each trivial difference amasses tremendously at the population level. Thus, we must conclude that health inequality is greater in the gigantic population than the small population. This conclusion strikes many people as absurd.

This example is not only an illustrative intellectual exercise. *The World Health Report 2000*, for example, ranked the health inequalities of its 191 member states. The smallest country was Niue, with only 2000 people, while the largest country was China, with 1,273,640,000 people (World Health Organization 2000a, 178). China was about 640,000 times bigger than Niue. With this difference in population size, any kind of sensitivity to the variable population size would end up with a non-trivial factor that determines the degree of health inequality.

I found that Temkin's proposal, in which inequality is worse in a larger population because there are more people suffering, has an intuitive appeal. In addition, empirical examinations of distributional concerns, albeit mostly in the income inequality context, have also revealed that the Population Principle may not be supported by people's perception of inequality as much as its predominant application suggests (Amiel and Cowell 1992; Harrison and Seidl 1994).

In summary, it would be worth questioning the Population Principle in the health context. But before abandoning it, we need to be clear about why we are interested in measuring health inequality and resolve the question raised by sensitivity to population size.

Subgroup Considerations

How should the judgment of inequality be sensitive to subgroup characteristics?

$$G_{overall} = G_{between\text{-}group} + G_{within\text{-}group} + G_{overlap}$$

SENSITIVITY TO THE SUBGROUP POPULATION SIZE
Among various subgroup considerations, the most frequently discussed is sensitivity to subgroup population size when measuring health inequality across groups (Illsley and Le Grand 1987; Wagstaff, Paci, and van Doorslaer 1991). Suppose that Population A and B have the same number of subgroups and exhibit the same pattern of inequality in each population. The size of the subgroups is different in Population A and B. Are the inequalities in Population A and B the same? Many researchers reasonably think not and believe that group-based health inequality measures should be sensitive to subgroup population size. Range measures are criticized for their insensitivity to subgroup population size (Illsley and Le Grand 1987; Wagstaff, Paci, and van Doorslaer 1991). They could lead to misleading results when applied to a comparison of populations with different subgroup population sizes. It is worth mentioning, however, that it is possible to use range measures sensitive to the subpopulation size. The World Bank, for example, used them to compare the health of those in the top 20% of income and those in the bottom 20% (World Bank 2006). Of course, 20% of the

population of 100 people is 20 people, and that of 1000 people is 200 people. The question of whether a health inequality measure should be sensitive to the absolute or proportional number of a subpopulation takes us back to the issue discussed in the previous section on sensitivity to the total population size.

SENSITIVITY TO SUBGROUP INEQUALITIES

An interesting subgroup consideration highly relevant to the health inequality context is how the overall inequality of a population measured by individual-based health inequality measures corresponds to inequalities of subgroups. A simple example will help explain this subgroup consideration. Suppose Population A and B have exactly the same distribution of health across individuals. By using such individual-based inequality measures as the Gini coefficient and the WHO health inequality index, one would obtain the same degree of health inequality in Population A and B. Now imagine that Population A is much like a society in the real world, where the rich are healthy while the poor sick, but Population B is an unusual society, where health is not correlated with income and wealth at all. With such a difference in health inequalities by subgroups, should one still conclude that Population A and B are the same in terms of health inequality? (for a graphic illustration of this example, see figure 1.2 in chapter 1).

As this example illustrates, even when we measure health inequality across individuals, we might wish to reflect subgroup inequality in total inequality. The WHO health inequality index has been widely criticized because it does not take any subgroup inequality into account.[29] But the other side of this criticism is that a group-based inequality measure cannot tell how much the grouping factor used in the analysis is accountable for the total health inequality in the population. Also, because it uses an aggregate measure, the group average, a group-based inequality measure neglects inequalities within groups.

The choice of the unit of analysis, individual or group, is often considered to be dichotomous, but it does not need to be (Wolfson and Rowe 2001). We can measure health inequalities across individuals and take subgroup inequality into consideration. One way to do so is with the subgroup decomposition technique, which is often used in income inequality measurement.

Income inequality research has developed a convenient view of the relationship between the total or overall inequality and subgroup inequalities. It is thought that total inequality of a population consists of inequalities within subgroups and inequalities between subgroups. To identify between-subgroup inequality, everyone within a subgroup is assumed to have the subgroup's mean level or the standardized level of the good of interest, in our case health. A property called subgroup consistency focuses on the relationship between total inequality and inequalities within subgroups. Another property called subgroup decomposability concerns whether total inequality can be decomposed into within-subgroup inequality and between- subgroup inequality. In the following, I discuss the desirability of these two properties in the health inequality context.

SUBGROUP CONSISTENCY[30]

Subgroup consistency states that the direction of the overall inequality must be responsive to the direction of inequalities within subgroups. Suppose our total population of interest is the Canadian population, and subpopulations are men and women. Subgroup consistency requires that if inequality among men stays the same but inequality among women increases, the overall inequality in Canada must increase.

Is this property what we wish for health inequality measurements? Perhaps not, because it imposes unrealistic constraint on our thinking about health inequality. Subgroup consistency is certainly useful from the policy perspective, as the consistency of inequality results send policy-makers a straightforward message whatever a population boundary may be. Yet it is unclear why we should expect that this property must hold for any grouping. Imagine that we are interested in health inequalities before and after the establishment of a universal health care system, or medicare, in Canada. We would want to know the change in overall health inequality as well as changes in health inequalities among the rich and the poor. Let us suppose that we found health inequality among the rich stayed the same but health inequality among the poor decreased. Using a subgroup-consistent inequality measure, we would obtain the result that overall health inequality in Canada decreased after the establishment of medicare. Income is one way to partition a population, but obviously there are many other characteristics with which we can partition a population, for example, rurality. Suppose further that we are also interested in changes in health inequalities within rural and urban communities. If income had a very strong relationship with health and could explain most of the variations in health, then the cause of health inequalities within the rural and urban communities may in fact primarily be the relationship between income and health. If rural communities were largely poor and urban communities rich, we would expect health inequality within rural communities to decrease but health inequality within urban communities to stay the same. But if the relationship between income and health was not that strong, then health inequalities within rural and urban communities would reflect something about living in rural or urban communities over and above the effect of income. It might be the case then health inequality within rural communities would stay the same but health inequality within urban communities would increase. As this example illustrates, subgroup consistency is perhaps too demanding a property.

A more interesting subgroup consideration in the health inequality context is perhaps inequalities between subgroups. Recall that the WHO health inequality index has been criticized as not paying attention to group characteristics important for health policy. An ideal health inequality measure would recognize the group contribution to overall inequality and incorporate that factor into the calculation of the overall inequality.

Constructing such a measure faces at least two difficult obstacles. First, such a measure inevitably violates one of the fundamental assumptions of individual-based inequality measures: inequality is judged only by the commodity of interest, in our case, health. With this assumption, we count, for example, eighty years of life as it is, whoever this eighty years of life belongs to, whether a mass murderer or a saint. Introducing other factors than health to the individual-based measurement of health inequality touches on the foundation of measurement construction. A second obstacle is the same as the problem for subgroup consistency: it is unrealistic to assume consistency for any grouping. We can, for example, reasonably imagine that health inequality between sexes becomes smaller, but at the same time, health inequality between urban and rural areas increases. In such a case, it is unclear how overall inequality should reflect these between-group inequalities going in the opposite directions.

SUBGROUP DECOMPOSITION

The discussion on subgroup consistency suggests that it is difficult to construct a health inequality measure that reflects our considerations of overall inequality as well as inequalities between subgroups. In what way can we reflect subgroup considerations into health inequality measurement? One way to do so is to decompose overall health inequality into inequalities within subgroups and between subgroups. In this way, an overall health inequality measure may judge that the two populations' inequalities are the same, but we have additional information on how much inequalities within and between subgroups account for the overall inequality.

In the income inequality literature, inequality measures whose overall inequality equals the sum of inequalities within and between subgroups are usually considered to be decomposable. They are sometimes called path independent inequality measures (Foster and Shneyerov 2000). Inequality measures known to satisfy this additive decomposability are the Generalized Entropy class measures (Sen 1997, 34–6). Although they are not traditionally applied to health distributions, Pradhan, Sahn, and Younger used the Theil entropy measure (one of the Generalized Entropy class measures) in their analysis of world health inequality (2003). Their choice of the inequality measure comes from their desire to decompose world health inequality into between- and within-country inequalities.

Subgroup decomposition of the Gini coefficient, a familiar inequality measure also used for health, has been studied extensively,[31] although it is not decomposable in the strict sense of path independence. Overall inequality measured by the Gini coefficient can be decomposed into inequalities within subgroups, inequalities between subgroups, and overlap. The Gini coefficient is decomposable in the same way as the path independent inequality measures only when there is no overlap. The Gini coefficient captures an additional aspect of subgroup inequalities, overlap, which is by definition neglected in the path independent inequality measures. While some scholars think that the overlap term does not offer any precise interpretation, others interpret it as a measure of the degree of stratification: a smaller degree of overlap suggests a higher degree of stratification (Warner 2001).[32] Yitzhaki and Lerman (1991) list three questions that the conventional individual- or group-based inequality measurement alone cannot address but that we can ask with subgroup decomposition. I introduce them in the health context:

- How much of overall health inequality comes from inequalities within subgroups, inequalities between subgroups, and the combination of stratification and inequalities within subgroups?
- To what extent do particular groups of interest occupy specific segments of the health distribution? What is the extent of stratification by the group with respect to health?

- Which way of grouping the population yields meaningful subgroups with respect to health ranking?

Further exploration is needed concerning the interpretation and use of the overlapping term in the health inequality context. Nonetheless, subgroup decomposition would be a promising strategy to simultaneously address many of our interests in health inequality. Indeed, recent studies have employed subgroup decomposition of the Concentration Index (Clarke, Gerdtham, and Connelly 2003; Wagstaff 2005). Unlike the Gini coefficient, the Concentration Index measures health inequality in relation to other goods, for example, income-related health inequality, and its subgroup decomposition uses one additional group characteristic. For example, income-related health inequality across all employment groups can be decomposed into income-related health inequality between and within employment groups and overlap. Simultaneous assessment of multiple aspects of health inequality is attractive. Yet overall inequality in subgroup decomposition of the Concentration Index is overall income-related health inequality, not overall inequality in the sense of subgroup decomposition of the Gini coefficient. Thus, subgroup decomposition of the Concentration Index cannot answer such a question as to what extent income-related health inequality explains overall health inequality.

4.5 Summary

In this chapter, we looked at five questions that arise in the process of summarizing a health distribution into one number. The preceding discussion suggests the following answers to the five questions as appropriate properties for a health inequality measure:

- Comparison: unless one has a particular interest in a specific person or group (e.g., the worst-off) or a certain norm (e.g., the basic level of health), everyone's health should be compared against everyone's health.
- Aggregation: greater weights should be attached towards the lower tail of the distribution, but no weight should be attached to differences.
- Sensitivity to the mean: one should adopt an intermediate inequality concept and judge that equal absolute addition reduces inequality while equal proportional increase increases inequality.
- Sensitivity to population size: one's measure of inequality should be

Table 4.3
The five questions and selected health inequality measures

Number of units = 2, range measures

	Ratio	Absolute difference	Shortfalls in achievement
Comparison	Often the worst-off x the best-off	Often the worst-off x the best-off	Group of focus x the norm
Aggregation	NA	NA	NA
Sensitivity to the mean	Scale invariant	Translation invariant	*
Sensitivity to the total population size	Insensitive	Insensitive	Insensitive
Subgroup considerations			
Sensitivity to the subpopulation size	Insensitive	Insensitive	Insensitive
Decomposability	NA	NA	NA

Number of units > 2, measures of health inequality in relation to other characteristics (e.g., socio-economic status)

	The Concentration Index	The generalized Concentration Index
Comparison	Everyone x everyone	Everyone x everyone
Aggregation	Weighted addition of health share Unweighted addition of differences	Weighted addition of health share Unweighted addition of differences
Sensitivity to the mean	Scale invariant	Translation invariant
Sensitivity to the total population size	Insensitive	Insensitive
Subgroup considerations		
Sensitivity to the subpopulation size	Sensitive	Sensitive
Decomposability	Possible**	Possible

Table 4.3 — (continued)

	Number of units > 2, measures of health inequality across individuals	
	The Gini coefficient	The WHO health inequality index
Comparison	Everyone x everyone	Everyone x everyone
Aggregation	Weighted addition of health share	Weighted addition of health share
	Unweighted addition of differences	Weighted addition of differences
Sensitivity to the mean	Scale invariant	Intermediate inequality
Sensitivity to the total population size	Insensitive	Insensitive
Subgroup considerations		
Sensitivity to the subpopulation size***	Can go either way	?
Decomposability	Possible	?

* Irregular. Both absolute addition and equal proportional increase reduce inequality

** Note the difference between subgroup decomposition of the Concentration Index and the Gini coefficient. When the Concentration Index measures income-related health inequality and decomposes it by employment, for example, income-related overall health inequality is decomposed into between and within employment groups and overlap. When the Gini coefficient is decomposed by employment, on the other hand, overall health inequality is decomposed into between and within employment groups and overlap.

*** For the Gini coefficient and the WHO health inequality index, whether subgroup decomposition is sensitive to the subpopulation size.

~~insensitive to population size, if the reason for measuring health~~
inequality is a concern for social justice.
• Subgroup considerations: (a) health inequality measures should be
  sensitive to subgroup population size, and (b) subgroup decomposability shows promising analytical advantages.

Throughout this chapter I have used the five popular health inequality
measures as examples. Table 4.3 summarizes how they respond to these
five questions. As it turns out, none of them satisfies all of these appropriate properties. How then should researchers choose among health
inequality measures available?

Researchers can decide the relative importance of the five questions
above and choose an available inequality measure that satisfies the
largest number of the most important properties. For example, among
the five popular health inequality measures, if one does not have interests in a specific person or group, or a certain norm, the Concentration
Index and the Gini coefficient appear to be most attractive satisfying all
desirable properties except sensitivity to the mean. One might then
wish to use the Concentration Index for measuring health inequality by
some characteristic, for example, income-related health inequality, and
the Gini coefficient for overall health inequality. The choice between
the Concentration Index and the Gini coefficient might also depend on
a particular kind of decomposition one is interested in. Using the Gini
coefficient, overall health inequality is decomposed by a group characteristic (e.g., employment), while using the Concentration Index,
overall health inequality related to some other characteristic (e.g.,
income-related health inequality) is decomposed by an additional
group characteristic (e.g., employment).

Alternatively, researchers can construct a health inequality measure
that satisfies appropriate properties, as Gakidou, Murray, and Frenk
(2001) attemped with the WHO health inequality index. However, how
the five questions relate to each other is an important issue that needs
further investigation. See appendix B for the relationship between questions of aggregation and sensitivity to the mean.

4.6 Framework Revisited

Now we are finishing part 1 of the book, and it will be useful to briefly
review what we have established so far before moving onto the empirical analyses in part 2. The previous two chapters and this chapter

Figure 4.6   Summary of part 1

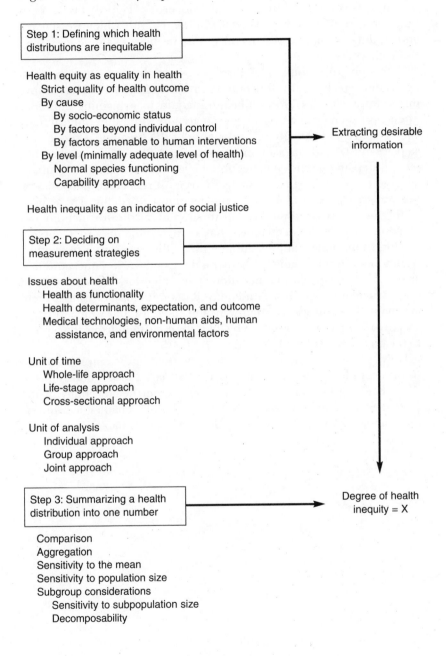

explained in detail a framework for measuring health inequity, that is, health inequality reflecting moral concern.[33] Figure 4.6 extends figure 1.4 in chapter 1, a skeletal framework with which we started, and summarizes major discussion points we have examined in these three chapters.

The framework consists of three steps. As the first step, we must determine which health distributions are inequitable. Chapter 2 introduced various perspectives on health inequity by explaining intuitions often expressed by health sciences researchers with philosophical theories of justice and equality. After defining health inequity, as the second step, we must decide measurement strategies. Chapter 3 focused on this second step and discussed issues about health, unit of time, and unit of analysis, emphasizing that these decisions must reflect moral considerations as well as data availability and technical feasibility. These steps enable us to extract desirable information about health inequity out of countless health inequalities that exist around us. To compare, examine, and understand health inequities, the final step is to quantify health inequity information. Chapter 4 discussed five key questions that arise in the process of quantification. The framework does not defend one particular view of health inequity. Rather, it emphasizes that there are many different ways to define health inequity, and whichever perspective we might take, we must be logically consistent from conception to measurement of health inequity.

How exactly then can this framework be used in the empirical analysis of health inequity? This is precisely what part 2 of the book aims to show. Keeping in mind the question of whether health equity in the United States improved between 1990 and 1995, chapter 5 connects the framework to an empirical demonstration, and chapter 6 shows the results of the empirical analyses.

PART TWO

Empirical Illustration

5 Bridging Concepts and Analysis

5.1 Overview

With the framework developed in part 1, we are now ready to move on to actual empirical analysis. In the chapters to follow, I show how we can apply the framework developed for measuring health inequity to empirical analysis. Adopting different perspectives on health equity from part 1, in part 2 I examine whether health equity improved in the United States between 1990 and 1995. Data used are the 1990 and 1995 U.S. National Health Interview Survey (NHIS). I analyse these same data sets according to different perspectives on health equity.

The primary objective of part 2 is to show the importance of logical consistency from conceptualization to measurement in health inequity analysis. Every measurement decision I make in health equity analyses in part 2 relates to discussions in part 1. The second objective is to highlight the possibility of drawing different conclusions regarding health inequity from the same data by examining these data from different perspectives on health equity, thereby highlighting the importance of selecting an appropriate health equity concept and measurement strategy for one's own purpose.

In addition to bridging concepts and empirical analysis, health inequity analyses in part 2 methodologically depart from previous empirical health inequity studies in the following three ways. First, I use a health status measure, the Health and Activity Limitation Index (HALex) (Erickson, Wilson, and Shannon 1995), as the health variable. Understanding health as a multi-purpose resource, chapter 3 advocated functionality as the focus of health in health inequity analysis, and this coincides with the focus of health status measures. None of the health status measures currently available is perfect, but their development is rapid and their use is growing. The future of health inequity analysis will evidently proceed with the development of health status measures. The HALex is the only health status measure currently available that can legitimately be applied to a nationally representative sample of the United States.

Second, I include the dead in the analysis of health inequity despite the use of a cross-sectional survey. A cross-sectional health survey usually only collects health information on the living and neglects the dead of the target population. Recognizing death as a health outcome, I would argue that analysis of the health of the living provides only partial information concerning health inequity in a population. However healthy the living population may be, if there were also a great proportion of deaths in the population, we may not be able to capture the true picture of health inequity merely by looking at the health of the living.[1] Accordingly, I assess health inequity not only by the living, but also whenever possible, including the dead.

Finally, I provide confidence intervals for the degree of health inequity estimated. Although a few pioneer studies exist,[2] drawing a statistical inference has yet to become a standard practice in health inequity analysis. Without a statistical inference, we cannot conclude with confidence whether health inequity has improved or worsened. Statisticians have developed bootstrap methods to overcome major difficulties in drawing a statistical inference for the degree of inequity estimated using data with a complex survey design, like the NHIS. The analyses in part 2 employ such methods.

For methodologically oriented readers, these features are, I believe, intriguing extensions of the bridge between concepts and empirical analysis of health equity. For those who lack advanced quantitative training, however, they might be too technical. As in part 1, in the following main text I limit mathematical notation as much as possible and explain quantitative methods in ordinary language as much as I can. Readers who are confused by the inclusion of the dead should feel free to restrict themselves to analyses of the living-only population. Analyses of the living-only population are the same as usual empirical studies using cross-sectional data. Should readers wish to skip technical materials altogether, I suggest they read only this section and section 5.3 in this chapter and section 6.2 in chapter 6. Those who wish to know technical materials in detail may refer to the appendices.

The plan of part 2 is as follows. Part 2 consists of two chapters:

chapter 5 discusses methods and chapter 6 presents empirical analyses. In section 5.2, I compose the building blocks necessary for examination of health inequity in the United States. I explain data and sample, of both the living and the dead, and the measurement of health, the HALex. Next, I discuss measurements of health inequity appropriate for analyses using these health inequity perspectives.[3] I then explain the unit of time used for analyses in part 2.

In section 5.3, as a preliminary analysis, I look at the average HALex in the United States in 1990 and 1995. It would be useful to get some sense of how healthy Americans were on average in terms of health status before examining how health status was distributed among Americans.

Using these building blocks, in chapter 6 I investigate whether health equity improved in the United States between 1990 and 1995 from different perspectives on health equity. All of the perspectives employed were introduced and discussed in part 1. First, I take the view of health inequality as an indicator of social justice. Second, I examine health inequity in the United States by race, sex and gender, income, or education. These examples show what conclusions we might draw regarding health equity if our interest was for a specific group characteristic. These analyses are based on our discussion in the section of the unit of analysis in chapter 3 that health inequity can be examined with a special interest in a specific group characteristic. These analyses also follow what is perhaps the most common way to assess health inequity, but I critique the ambiguity of analysing health inequity in such a way.

Third, I adopt the view of health inequity as health inequality caused by socio-economic status (SES). As discussed in chapter 2, two types of philosophical justification are possible to support the view of health inequity as health inequality caused by SES: the Rawlsian difference principle (Rawls 1971) and Walzer's view of dominance as unjust (Walzer 1983). Accordingly, I examine health equity in the United States based on these two views. Although they share the umbrella category of health inequity as health inequality caused by SES, I show that analytical strategies differ.

Finally, I employ the view of health equity as satisfying the minimally adequate level of health. Based on our discussion in chapter 3, for this I use Nussbaum's version of the Capability approach (Nussbaum 2000). As we saw in chapters 2 and 3, none of the philosophical theories applied in this chapter is flawless. Yet in the following, I assume that they are strong enough to provide a basis for empirical analysis of health inequity. Section 6.2 concludes part 2 with discussion.

5.2 Building Blocks

In this section I compose building blocks necessary for empirical analyses from different perspectives on health equity in chapter 6. Questions addressed in this section might appear to be ordinary measurement questions, for example, what measurements of health and health inequity would be appropriate? Should we stratify results by age group? We can make such measurement decisions based on convenience. Yet in part 1, I argued that there are various reasons why we choose one strategy over another due to our value of health and its distribution. This section shows connections between concepts and measurement strategies.

Data and Sample

Data for the living come from the 1990 and 1995 National Health Interview Survey (NHIS).[4] This cross-sectional survey uses a stratified multi-stage probability design, yielding a nationally representative sample of the civilian non-institutionalized U.S. population with a response rate of over 95% by face-to-face household interview. Surrogate information is obtained for children younger than seventeen years of age and persons absent at the time of the interview. Observations are excluded if an answer to a question necessary to construct the HALex is missing (0.5% missing in 1990, 1.2% missing in 1995). The sample size of the living for the following analyses is 119,003 (1990) and 101,277 (1995).

A cross-sectional survey only collects information on the living. To assess health inequity in the entire population, the information of the dead needs to be supplemented. Using life tables for the U.S. men and women (Anderson 1999; National Center for Health Statistics 1997), I imputed 1007 dead for the 1990 data and 747 for the 1995 data. See appendix C for details of the dead imputation method.

Table 5.1 shows the unweighted number of observations by age group, sex, race, education, income, and poverty in 1990 and 1995 both for the living and the dead. I use weighted data for all analyses in the following unless otherwise stated.

Measurement of Health: Health and Activity Limitation Index (HALex)

JUSTIFICATION
The measurement of health I am going to use in all health inequity analyses in part 2 is the Health and Activity Limitation Index (HALex),

Table 5.1
Basic description of sample, 1990 and 1995

	The living				The living + the dead			
	1990		1995		1990		1995	
	N	%	N	%	N	%	N	%
All ages	119,003	100	101,277	100	120,010	100	102,024	100
Age, years								
0–14	27,822	23.4	24,661	24.4	27,848	23.2	24,679	24.2
15–24	16,289	13.7	13,510	13.3	16,305	13.6	13,522	13.3
25–44	37,886	31.8	31,435	31.0	37,953	31.6	31,489	30.9
45–64	22,487	18.9	19,834	19.6	22,732	18.9	19,973	19.6
65+	14,519	12.2	11,837	11.7	15,173	12.6	12,361	12.1
Women	62,173	52.2	53,011	52.3	62,675	52.2	53,364	52.3
Race								
White	97,290	81.8	83,527	82.5				
Black	17,886	15.0	13,629	13.5				
Other	3,827	3.2	4,121	4.1				
Education (25+ years old)								
Less than 12 years	16,577	22.4	13,446	21.6				
12 years	28,386	38.3	22,713	36.5				
13–15 years	13,822	18.7	12,304	19.8				
16 years or more	15,289	20.6	13,704	22.0				
All years	74,074	100	62,167	100				
Income								
Less than $15,000	21,753	21.9	17,417	20.5				
$15,000–$24,999	19,254	19.4	15,724	18.5				
$25,000–$34,999	16,645	16.8	13,417	15.8				
$35,000–$49,999	18,813	19.0	15,569	18.3				
$50,000 or more	22,778	23.0	22,777	26.8				
All income	99,243	100	84,904	100				
Poverty								
At or above poverty threshold	94,842	87.6	77,690	84.4				
Below poverty threshold	13,374	12.4	14,379	15.6				
Total	108,216	100	92,069	100				

*In both 1990 and 1995, all living observations for which the HALex values can be assigned have information on sex and race. In 1990, education has 1.1% missing values, income 16.6%, and poverty 9.1%, and in 1995, education has 1.5% missing values, income 16.2%, and poverty 9.2%. Because the dead are imputed based only on age and sex, they do not have information on race, education, income, and poverty.

that is, the health-related quality of life part of the Years of Healthy Life (YHL) (Erickson, Wilson, and Shannon 1995). The HALex is a health status measure that expresses health states by numbers between zero (dead) and one (full health). In our appreciation of health, we value both living long and living well. The traditional concern of health goes to the former value, while health status measures attempt to capture the latter value, the health-related quality of life that goes along with the length of life.

The choice of a health status measure as the measurement of health for health inequity analysis is consistent with the discussion of health measurement in chapter 3. Understanding health as a multi-purpose resource, in chapter 3 I advocated functionality and general symptoms as the dimension of health that we should measure in health inequity analysis. This understanding of health is fundamental for all perspectives on health equity introduced in part 1, thus, for health inequity analyses in part 2 using them, the best dimension of health is functionality and general symptoms. In addition, I also showed in chapter 3 that health inequity analysis and health status measures look at the same dimension of health. Therefore, the use of a health status measure as the measurement of health in health inequity analysis is reasonable.

CONSTRUCTION
The HALex was created for the purpose of assisting one of the three goals of *Healthy People 2000*: increasing the span of healthy life for Americans (U.S. Department of Health and Human Services 1991). The HALex was developed to monitor both quality and quantity aspects of the health of the population. Constructing a health status measure often requires an explicit value assessment, yet there was no resource to conduct such a value assessment. Erickson and her colleagues then based a new measurement on existing information, the life table of the U.S. population and morbidity information from the NHIS (1995). Its construct and validity were later evaluated and confirmed (Erickson 1998). Although the HALex shortcuts complicated issues in the value assignment procedure, the HALex is the only health status measure that was specifically designed for, and can legitimately be applied to, a representative sample of the U.S. population. Methodology to assign a value to a health status has been extensively studied,[5] but it is beyond the scope of this book to look further into this issue.

The HALex combines two types of questions collected in the NHIS, one assessing activity limitation and the other measuring self-perceived

Table 5.2
The HALex scores

| Activity limitation | Single attribute score | Perceived health status | | | | | |
		Excellent 1.00	Very good 0.85	Good 0.70	Fair 0.30	Poor 0.00	Dead
Not limited	1.00	1.00	0.92	0.84	0.63	0.47	
Limited in performing other activities	0.75	0.87	0.79	0.72	0.52	0.38	
Limited in performing major activities	0.65	0.81	0.74	0.67	0.48	0.34	
Unable to perform major activity	0.40	0.68	0.62	0.55	0.38	0.25	
Limited in instrumental activities of daily living (IADL)	0.20	0.57	0.51	0.45	0.29	0.17	
Limited in activities of daily living (ADL)	0.00	0.47	0.41	0.36	0.21	0.10	
Dead							0.00

Source: Erickson, Wilson, and Shannon (1995).

health (Erickson, Wilson, and Shannon 1995). The activity limitation questions create six categories: (1) not limited, (2) limited in other activities, (3) limited in major activity, (4) unable to perform major activity, (5) unable to perform instrumental activities of daily living, and (6) unable to perform activities of daily living. Self-perceived health is in five categories: excellent, very good, good, fair, and poor.[6] These two items together make up a matrix of thirty combinations (table 5.2).

Assignment of a score to each of these thirty combinations took three steps. Developers of the HALex first assigned a score for each of the six levels of activity limitation and the five levels of self-perceived health ('Single attribute score' in table 5.2), using a mathematical technique called correspondence analysis. Correspondence analysis belongs to a family of multidimensional scaling, a technique creating a scale for a concept with multiple dimensions, for example, health consisting of mobility, sensory apprehension, cognition, emotion, and pain, or social support consisting of informational, emotional, and practical support. Correspondence analysis finds the best simultaneous representation of two domains, activity limitation and self-perceived health in the case of the HALex, by maximizing the correlation between them.

The simplest correspondence analysis applies to a two-way cross-tabulation, as in the case for the HALex, activity limitation and self-perceived health. One can assign a score for each of the six levels of activity limitation by weighted least-squares where each of the six levels of activity limitation is weighted by its frequency divided by the total frequency of the six levels, and distances between each of the six levels are measured by the chi-square distance. To measure the distance between 'not limited' and 'limited in performing other activities' in activity limitation, for example, correspondence analysis uses the chi-square distance between these two categories by examining how people in these two categories differ with respect to the five levels of self-perceived health. Developers of the HALex conducted separate correspondence analysis for each of several different five-year age groups and different years of the NHIS. Based on the analyses, they assigned single attribute scores for each of the two domains as listed in table 5.2 that maximize the correlation between activity limitation and self-perceived health in all age groups.[7]

Next, the developers of the HALex made the following assumptions. They assumed that the score for the health state with no activity limitation and excellent self-perceived health is 1.00, and the score for the health state with limited activities of daily living and poor self-perceived health is 0.10. In addition, they assumed that a health state with limited activities of daily living and excellent self-perceived health is equally bad as the health state with no activity limitation and poor self-perceived health. Based on another health status measure, the Health Utilities Index Mark I, they assigned the score of 0.47 for these two health states.

Finally, using the scores assigned for each level of activity limitation and self-perceived health, and the four scores based on the assumptions described above, the developers of the HALex calculated scores for the rest of the twenty-six health states. The formula of this calculation is based on multiattribute utility theory. Multiattribute utility theory extends the traditional expected utility theory, a theory of rational decision making under uncertainty, by adding an independence assumption. The developers of the HALex, in particular, assumed mutual utility independence, that is, health domains other than self-perceived health and activity limitation (for example, pain, emotion, or hearing) have no effect on the HALex score. For example, the HALex score for the health state with limited activities of daily living and excellent self-perceived health is 0.47 regardless of the existence of pain or emotional or hearing problems. Due to this mutual utility independence assumption, the developers of the HALex used a multiplicative function for calculating the HALex scores.[8]

Erickson later evaluated and confirmed the construct validity of the HALex (1998). For the following health inequality analysis, I assign a HALex score to each observation in the 1990 and 1995 data. In addition, for the dead imputed I assign a HALex score of zero.

Measurements of Health Inequity

Recall the five key questions discussed in chapter 4 that arise when summarizing health inequity information into one number. The discussion in chapter 4 concluded the following answers to these questions as favourable properties for the measurement of health inequity:

- Comparison: unless one has a particular interest in a specific person or group (for example, the worst-off) or a certain norm (for example, the basic level of health), everyone's health should be compared against everyone's health.
- Aggregation: greater weights should be attached towards the lower tail of the distribution, but no weight should be attached to differences.
- Sensitivity to the mean: one should adopt an intermediate inequality concept and judge that equal absolute addition reduces inequality while equal proportional increase increases inequality.
- Sensitivity to population size: one's measure of inequality should be insensitive to population size, if the reason for measuring health inequality is a concern for social justice.
- Subgroup considerations: (a) health inequality measures should be sensitive to subgroup population size, and (b) subgroup decomposability shows promising analytical advantages.

When one does not have a particular interest in a specific person or group, or a certain norm, among popular inequality measures used for health inequity analysis, the Concentration Index and the Gini coefficient satisfy the greatest number of these properties (all but sensitivity to the mean). These measures have two primary differences. First, the Concentration Index measures health inequality by some characteristic, for example, income, gender, or race, while the Gini coefficient measures overall health inequity. Using subgroup decomposition, it is still possible to look at health inequity by some characteristic with the Gini coefficient. As discussed in chapter 4, subgroup decomposition of the Gini coefficient can suggest how much of overall health inequity comes from between and within group inequity and overlap.

The second primary difference between the Concentration Index and the Gini coefficient is the way in which subgroup decomposition is done. Suppose that we use the Concentration Index for measuring health inequity by education. If we decompose this education-related health inequity by one additional characteristic, say, gender, we can see how much of education-related health inequity can be explained by inequity within men and women, inequity between mean and women, and overlap. The Gini coefficient, on the other hand, measures overall health inequity. If we decompose overall health inequity by education, we can obtain information on how much of overall health inequity comes from inequity within each of education groups, inequity between education groups, and overlap. The attractiveness of this difference in subgroup decomposition of the Concentration Index and the Gini co-efficient depends on the purposes of a study.

Among perspectives on health equity (based on which I conduct empirical analysis in the following), the view of health inequality as an indicator of social justice, the view of health inequity as health inequality associated with a specific group characteristic, and the view of health inequity as health inequality associated with socio-economic status (based on Walzer's view of dominance as unjust) do not have a special interest in a particular person or group, or a norm. I use the Gini coefficient as the measurement of health inequity for these perspectives. The view of health inequality as an indicator of social justice focuses on overall health inequality, thus, based on the discussion in chapter 4, the Gini coefficient is a suitable measure. Other perspectives examine health inequality with some other characteristic, and, following the conclusions of chapter 4, the Concentration Index and the Gini coefficient (using subgroup decomposition) are candidate measures. With my interest in exploring subgroup decomposition of the Gini coefficient, I opt for the Gini coefficient for these perspectives, too.

Other equity perspectives on health equity, the view of health inequity as health inequality caused by socio-economic status (based on the Rawlsian difference principle) pays special attention to the worst-off group, and the view of health equity as satisfying the minimally adequate level of health is concerned about a specific norm of the minimally adequate level of health. Because of the conceptual similarity, I apply a poverty measure, the Foster-Greer-Thorbecke measure (Foster, Greer, and Thorbecke 1984) to the view of health equity as satisfying the minimally adequate level of health. For the analysis adopting the Rawlsian difference principle, I simply look at the health of the worst-off group among the living population.

Below I introduce the Gini coefficient and the Foster-Greer-Thorbecke measure.

THE GINI COEFFICIENT

Definition and Justification   The Gini coefficient (G) is defined as

$$G = \frac{1}{2} \sum_{i=1}^{n} \sum_{j=1}^{n} \frac{|y_i - y_j|}{n^2 \mu} \; ,$$

where the target population holds n people, y_i is the HALex score of individual i, y_j is the HALex score of individual j, and the average HALex in the population is μ (for an explanation of the Gini coefficient using a graph, see appendix A). The Gini coefficient takes a value between zero (perfectly equal) and one (most unequal).

The Gini coefficient satisfies all five desirable properties for the measurement of health inequity except sensitivity to the mean. The desirable property of sensitivity to the mean concluded in chapter 4 is the intermediate inequality concept, that is, judging the equal absolute addition reduces inequality while the equal proportional increase makes inequality bigger. The Gini coefficient does not use this intermediate inequality concept; instead, it is scale invariant, judging that the equal absolute addition reduces inequality while the equal proportional change does not affect inequality.

If one were eager to seek a measurement of health inequity satisfying all desirable properties, it would be possible to modify the Gini coefficient so as to introduce the intermediate inequality concept. But such an attempt comes with considerable cost. The Gini coefficient has been studied extensively, including its decomposability and statistical inference.[9] If one modified the Gini coefficient, one would not be able to benefit from these studies. Moreover, the five key questions arising in the process of summarizing a distribution into one number in a complex way relate to each other (see appendix B). Modification of one property must be carefully examined in relation to other properties. Given these considerations, I use the Gini coefficient without any modification in the following analyses.(See appendix D1 regarding the difference between the degrees of inequity obtained by the scale and translation invariant Gini coefficient. See appendix D2 regarding technical issues that arise in applying the Gini coefficient to the HALex.)

Statistical Inference for the Gini Coefficient   Health inequity analyses using the Gini coefficient in part 2 encounter two sets of challenges in the attempt to draw a statistical inference for the degree of inequity estimated. The first is due to the complex survey design of the NHIS. The second comes from the use of the Gini coefficient as the measurement of health inequity. Unlike a simple statistic, for example, the mean, the Gini coefficient is a non-linear function and bounded between zero and one, which makes it difficult to use asymptotic theory.

I seek the solution in the bootstrap method. The bootstrap is a simulation method using only data at hand, and with a few assumptions, it can provide a statistical inference for any statistic, including the Gini coefficient. To account for the complex survey design of the NHIS, I use a bootstrap method modified for survey data with complex design: the two-stage With-Replacement Bootstrap (BWR).[10] To obtain reliable confidence intervals, I repeat the simulation process 2000 times. (For a detailed explanation of a bootstrap method, see appendix D3.)

Subgroup Decomposition of the Gini Coefficient   In chapters 3 and 4, I suggested that the choice of the unit of analysis, individual or group, is not necessarily dichotomous, and that we can simultaneously measure health inequity across individuals and groups of individuals. Subgroup decomposition of the Gini coefficient is one way to do so. Let me explain the decomposition technique with the help of illustrations.

Customarily, health inequity by group, for example, racial or income group, is examined by comparing the average health between groups (figure 5.1a). But it is often questionable whose value is the average value, especially when, as is often the case for the distribution of the HALex, the shape of a distribution does not follow a normal distribution. Figures 5.1b and 5.1c illustrate that the same mean difference in health by group in figure 5.1a can come from different shapes of health distribution. Note that the degree of overlap between the two groups in figure 5.1b is substantially smaller than that of figure 5.1c. Despite the same absolute mean difference, the extent of group stratification or isolation with respect to health is greater in figure 5.1b than figure 5.1c. When looking at differences in the HALex between groups in the fol-

Figure 5.1   Mean difference, small overlap, and big overlap*

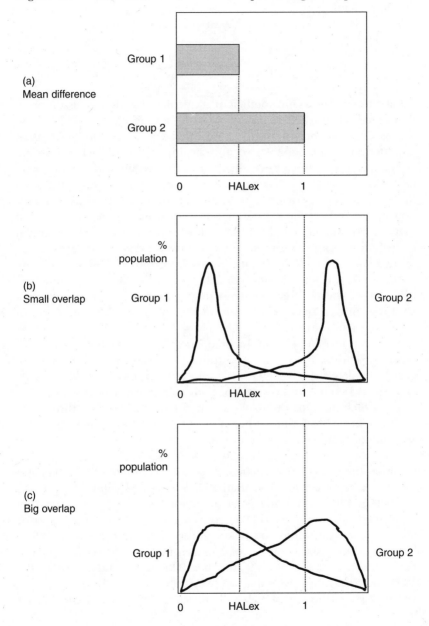

* These figures are not based on actual distributions and are used only for illustrative purposes.

lowing analyses, I add this overlap information to the conventional absolute mean.[11]

The overlap can be examined by subgroup decomposition of the Gini coefficient (G):

$$G_{overall} = G_{between\text{-}group} + G_{within\text{-}group} + G_{overlap}.$$

The between-group Gini coefficient is calculated under the assumption that everybody's health in a subgroup is its average health. The within-group Gini coefficient is first calculated for each subgroup, then weighted by population share and health share of each subgroup. $G_{within\text{-}group}$ in the equation is the sum of the within-group Gini coefficients for all subgroups. The overlap term captures the area shared by health distributions of subgroups and can be understood as stratification or isolation. When subgroups do not overlap, the overlap term equals zero. In analysing health inequity by group, I look at how much contribution (expressed in percentage) this overlap term makes to the overall Gini coefficient. Health equity by group is better when the overlap term makes a greater contribution to the Gini coefficient and the absolute mean difference between groups is smaller. (See appendix D4 for a more formal explanation of the subgroup decomposition of the Gini coefficient.)

I use sex, race, education, income, and poverty as subgroup characteristics for decomposition. I postpone discussion of which of these group characteristics is used exactly for what purpose in health inequity analysis and limit attention here to their basic information as variables. Sex is a dichotomous variable: male and female. Race has three categories: White, Black, and other. Education is applied only for those who are 25 years of age or older and has four categories: (1) less than 12 years of education, (2) 12 years, (3) 13–15 years, and (4) 16 years or more. Income is family income all sources combined before tax and has five categories: (1) less than $15,000, (2) $15,000–$24,999, (3) $25,000–$34,999, (4) $35,000–$44,999, and (5) $50,000 or more (all figures are in U.S. dollars). Poverty is a dichotomous variable: at or above poverty threshold and below poverty threshold. This variable is based on family size, number of children under 18 years of age, and family income using the 1989 (for the 1990 NHIS) and 1994 (for the 1995 NHIS) poverty levels derived from 1990 and 1995 Current Population Survey (Bureau of Labor Statistics and Bureau of the Census 2001).

THE FOSTER-GREER-THORBECKE (FGT) MEASURE

Definition and Justification   In one of the health inequity analyses below, I adopt the view of health equity as satisfying the minimally adequate level of health. The similarity is obvious between measuring poverty and measuring health inequity from the perspective of satisfying the minimally adequate level of health. Analysis of health inequity using this perspective applies many of the measurement strategies in the poverty measurement literature.

Sen lists the following three points as distinctive characteristics of poverty measurements (1997, 168–70):

1 The head-count ratio
2 The income-gap index
3 A measure of distribution of incomes among the poor

Most poverty measures use one of these characteristics or combine two or three. Poverty measures using characteristic (1) are most popular among policy-makers. They ask how many (or proportion of) people are poor. Measures using characteristic (2) are the second most popular and capture the 'depth' of the poverty: They ask how far off the poor are from the threshold. Sen is critical of poverty measures using only these two characteristics as they ignore the distribution of income among the poor. He suggests that a poverty measure will satisfy all of these three characteristics.

These arguments in poverty measurement are directly applicable to measurement of health inequity using the idea of the minimally adequate level of health. In the health context, the poverty threshold is the minimally adequate level of health, and the 'poor' are people whose health is below the minimally adequate level of health. We would wish to know how many (or proportion of) people are below the minimally adequate level of health, how far off they are from that level, and how health is distributed below that line.

Popular poverty measures that satisfy all of these three characteristics are the Foster-Greer-Thorbecke (FGT) measure and the Sen-Shorrocks-Thon (SST) measure.[12] By comparing the FGT measure with the SST measure using the framework developed in chapter 4, I opt for the FGT measure for the analysis adopting the view of health equity as satisfying the minimally adequate level of health. (See appendix E2 for details of the comparison between the FGT and SST measures.)

The FGT measure is defined as follows:

$$P_\alpha = \frac{1}{N} \sum_{i=1}^{n} \left(\frac{z - y_i}{z} \right)^\alpha,$$

where N is the total population, and n is the total number of those who below the threshold, z. We line up people from the sickest to the healthiest, and y_i is health of individual i. $z - y_i$ only applies to those below the threshold, thus suggesting the shortfalls of health of the ith individual. α is a measure of the sensitivity to the health gap. The larger the α is, the more weight is assigned to sicker people below the threshold.

When $\alpha = 0$, the FGT measure is the head-count ratio and measures the proportion of people below the threshold in the population. The FGT measure ($\alpha = 0$) takes values between 0 and 1, suggesting, respectively, no one is below the threshold and everyone is below the threshold.

When $\alpha = 1$, the FGT measure is the health-gap index and measures the average shortfall of people below the threshold over the whole population, expressed as a ratio to the threshold. It asks what proportion of the minimally adequate level of health people below that level lack on average over the whole population. When the FGT measure ($\alpha = 1$) equals to 0.15, for example, the average health gap, when spreading both above and below the threshold, is equivalent to 15% of the value of the minimally adequate level of health. The FGT measure ($\alpha = 1$) takes values between 0 and 1, suggesting, respectively, no shortfall at all (that is, no one is below the minimally adequate level) and 100% shortfall (that is, everyone in the population is dead, and therefore, everyone is below the minimally adequate level of health). The FGT measure ($\alpha = 1$) does not take account of how many people are below the line, but on average how far off those who below the line are.

When $\alpha = 2$, the FGT measure is the squared health-gap index, a weighted sum of health gaps with the weight of a proportionate health gap itself. The FGT measure ($\alpha = 2$) is the combination of the head-count ratio, the health gap index, and a measure of distribution of health below the threshold, therefore, sensitive to the inequality among those who below the threshold. The FGT measure ($\alpha = 2$) takes values between 0 and 1, suggesting, respectively, that no one is below the threshold and that everyone is dead, therefore, is below the threshold. Smaller values between 0 and 1 suggest a greater achievement of the minimally adequate level of health but do not provide intuitive interpretation like the FGT measure ($\alpha = 0$) and ($\alpha = 1$).

In the following health inequity analysis adopting the perspective of health equity as satisfying the minimally adequate level of health, I use the FGT measure ($\alpha = 2$) as the measurement of health inequity. To compensate for the lack of intuitive interpretation of this measure, I also provide results of the FGT measure ($\alpha = 0$) and the FGT measure ($\alpha = 1$). These three results together help us understand how large a proportion of people are below the threshold ($\alpha = 0$), how far off those people are from the threshold ($\alpha = 1$), and what is the degree of health inequity taking the distribution of health among people below the threshold into account in addition to these two considerations ($\alpha = 2$). (For mathematical notations of the FGT measure when equals to zero, one, and two, see appendix E1.)

Decomposition   In chapters 3 and 4, I argued that the perspective of health equity as satisfying the minimally adequate level of health is the only equity perspective introduced in this project whose concept strongly supports the individual as the unit of analysis. Even in this perspective, decomposition by subpopulation group will be useful for policy-making. The FGT measure (P) can be decomposed by subgroup population as follows:

$$P_{total} = \frac{1}{N_{total}} \sum \left(P_{within\text{-}group} \cdot N_{group} \right).$$

Total health inequity is the sum of within-group health inequity weighted by the population share. In other words, by decomposing health inequity by subpopulation group, we can know health inequity within each group, and, with the information on the population share of each group, we can assess the impact of health inequity reduction policy.

In the following analysis of health equity with the idea of the minimally adequate level of health, I decompose the FGT measure whenever deemed meaningful. Group characteristics used for the decomposition of the FGT measure are the same as those of the Gini coefficient (sex, race, education, income, and poverty). (See appendix E3 for mathematical notations for decomposition of the FGT measure.)

Statistical Inference for the Foster-Greer-Thorbecke (FGT) Measure   As for inequality measures in general, the importance of statistical inference for poverty measures has increasingly been pointed out.[13] I therefore draw a statistical inference for the Foster-Greer-Thorbecke (FGT) Measure, using the linearization method. (See appendix E4 for details.)

Unit of Time

In the section of the unit of time in chapter 3, I advocated the life-stage approach as the desirable consideration of the unit of time in health inequity analysis. Understanding health as a multi-purpose resource whose value is likely to vary at different stages of life, I argued that health inequity is most reasonably assessed within each age group. Accordingly, in analyses in part 2, I use the following age groups: 0–14, 15–24, 25–44, 45–64, 65+ years old. These five age groups reflect epidemiological profiles as humans and developmental stages as a person. Recall that one of the fundamental values of health as a multi-purpose resource supports the life-stage approach. Because all perspectives on health equity employed in this chapter share this fundamental value of health, all health equity analyses in part 2 favour the life-stage approach.[14]

The discussion in chapter 3 suggested the conceptual appeal of the life-stage approach. Yet, with cross-sectional data in hand, in epidemiological study it is common to look at a snapshot picture of all ages combined. Is this a problem? I discussed in chapter 3 that comparison of health inequities of cross-sectional snapshots could be a problem if the age structures of the populations compared were different. Health is largely determined by age, but we have yet to come to a consensus as to whether health inequality associated with age is inequitable. To rephrase, one could reasonably assess health inequity of all ages combined if the target populations had a similar age structure.

To see whether health inequity of all ages in 1990 and 1995 can be reasonably compared, let us once again look at table 5.1 and see the age compositions of 1990 and 1995 populations. For the living population and the population of the living and the dead combined, age compositions appear to be quite similar in 1990 and 1995. This similarity suggests that comparison of health inequities of 1990 and 1995 populations of all ages would not suffer from the issue of age as a cause of inequity. In health inequity analyses in the following, I accordingly examine health inequity of all ages combined as well as by age group.

With data, the measurement of health, measurements of health inequity, and considerations for the unit of time, we now have sufficient tools to examine health inequity. As a preliminary to health equity analyses, in the following section let us first look at how healthy Americans were on average in terms of health status in 1990 and 1995.

Table 5.3
The average HALex and life expectancy in the United States in 1990 and 1995 by sex and age

	Both sexes (95% CI)	Male (95% CI)	Female (95% CI)
Life expectancy, years			
1990	75.4	71.8	78.8
1995	75.8	72.5	78.9
The Average HALex, the living + the dead			
All ages			
1990	0.87	0.86	0.87
1995	0.87	0.86	0.85
The Average HALex, the living			
All ages			
1990	0.87 (0.87, 0.88)	0.88 (0.88, 0.88)	0.87 (0.86, 0.87)
1995	0.87 (0.86, 0.87)	0.87 (0.87, 0.88)	0.86 (0.86, 0.86)
0–14 years			
1990	0.93 (0.93, 0.93)	0.93 (0.93, 0.93)	0.94 (0.93, 0.94)
1995	0.93 (0.93, 0.93)	0.93 (0.92, 0.93)	0.94 (0.93, 0.94)
15–24 years			
1990	0.92 (0.92, 0.92)	0.93 (0.92, 0.93)	0.91 (0.91, 0.91)
1995	0.91 (0.91, 0.91)	0.92 (0.92, 0.92)	0.91 (0.90, 0.91)
25–44 years			
1990	0.90 (0.90, 0.90)	0.90 (0.90, 0.91)	0.89 (0.89, 0.89)
1995	0.89 (0.88, 0.89)	0.90 (0.89, 0.90)	0.88 (0.88, 0.88)
45–64 years			
1990	0.82 (0.82, 0.83)	0.83 (0.82, 0.83)	0.82 (0.81, 0.82)
1995	0.81 (0.81, 0.82)	0.82 (0.82, 0.83)	0.81 (0.80, 0.81)
65+ years			
1990	0.73 (0.72, 0.74)	0.74 (0.74, 0.75)	0.72 (0.71, 0.73)
1995	0.73 (0.72, 0.73)	0.73 (0.73, 0.74)	0.72 (0.71, 0.73)

5.3 How Healthy Were Americans on Average in 1990 and 1995?

Overall HALex in 1990 and 1995

Table 5.3 presents the average HALex, its 95% Confidence Intervals (CI), and life expectancy (National Center for Health Statistics 1994; 1998) of the U.S. population in 1990 and 1995 by sex and age group. The average HALex is reported both for the living U.S. population and the U.S. population of the living and the dead combined. Between 1990 and 1995, overall Americans' health slightly improved in terms of the length

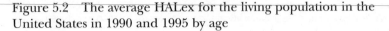

Figure 5.2   The average HALex for the living population in the
United States in 1990 and 1995 by age

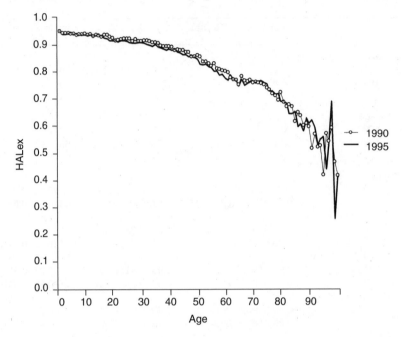

of life (0.4-year increase for both sexes, 0.7-year increase for men, and
0.1-year increase for women), but not the average HALex. During these
years, among the living U.S. population, the average HALex for both
sexes (0.87 in both years), men (0.88 in 1990, 0.87 in 1995), and women
(0.87 in 1990, 0.86 in 1995) of these two years were not statistically significantly different at the 5% level. Among the U.S. population of the
living and the dead combined, the average HALex decreased by 0.01 for
both sexes and 0.01 for women and stayed the same for men.

The HALex by Age Group

Figure 5.2 suggests that the decline in the HALex between 1990 and
1995 was not consistent at every age. Table 5.3 shows that the average
HALex for both sexes was lower among 15–24 and 25–44 year olds in
1995 than 1990 ($p < 0.05$). Differences between the average HALex in
1990 and 1995 within other age groups were not statistically significant

Figure 5.3   The average HALex for the living population in the
United States in 1990 by sex and age

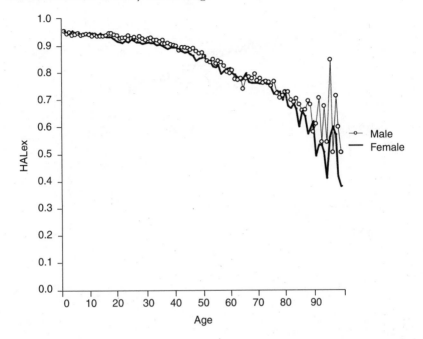

at the 5% level. Fluctuation of the HALex at older ages is likely to be
due to the small number of observations.

The HALex by Sex

Life expectancy for women has always been higher than men in the
United States, as in most of the countries in the world. The healthiness
of American women measured by the length of life, however, does not
appear to translate to health status. Figures 5.3 and 5.4 indicate that.
Table 5.3 shows that in both 1990 and 1995 overall women's HALex was
lower than men's (0.01 difference, p<0.05 both in 1990 and 1995). This
was true in all age groups, except among 0–14 year olds both in 1990
and 1995, 45–64 year olds in 1990, and 65+ year olds in 1995.

   Why is women's HALex almost always lower than men's? To investigate this question, I look at the distributions of two components of the
HALex, self-perceived health and activity limitation (data not shown).

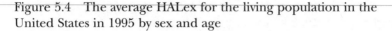

Figure 5.4   The average HALex for the living population in the United States in 1995 by sex and age

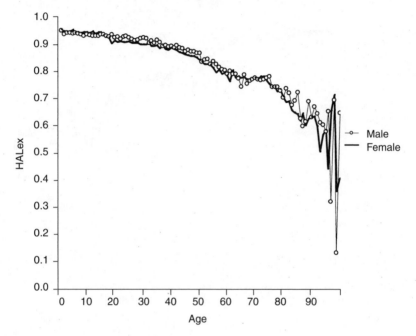

The Pearson Chi-square tests suggest that differences between men and women in reporting self-perceived health and activity limitation are statistically significant at the 5% level in both 1990 and 1995. Judging from the magnitude of these differences, they are likely to be driven more by the difference in self-perceived health than in activity limitation.[15]

Summary

The results above suggest that the length of life and the health-related quality of life capture different aspects of health. Between 1990 and 1995 in the United States, life expectancy (length of life) improved but the HALex (health-related quality of life) did not improve. Women tend to live longer but with lower health-related quality of life than men. Analyses of the HALex provide additional information to the length of life.

Figure 5.5   The HALex distribution for the living and the dead
populations in the United States in 1990

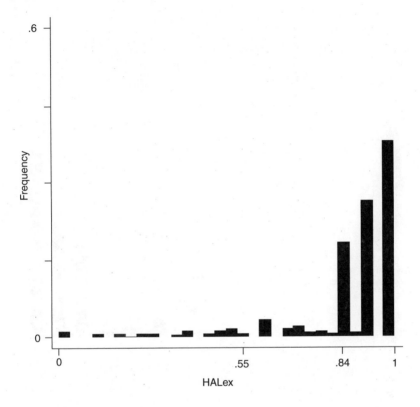

Let me emphasize again that the analyses in this chapter focused on
the average. In other words, in this chapter I assessed how healthy
Americans were *on average* in 1990 and 1995. This is one way, and often
a quite useful way, to look at the health of a population. But the average
value is by definition one number from a population. What of the distribution of health – how health was distributed within the United
States in 1990 and 1995? Figures 5.5 and 5.6 illustrate the distribution
of the HALex of the U.S. population of the living and the dead combined in 1990 and 1995. What do we make of these figures? How equitable are these distributions of health? These are precisely the questions
I will ask in the next chapter.

Figure 5.6   The HALex distribution for the living and the dead
populations in the United States in 1995

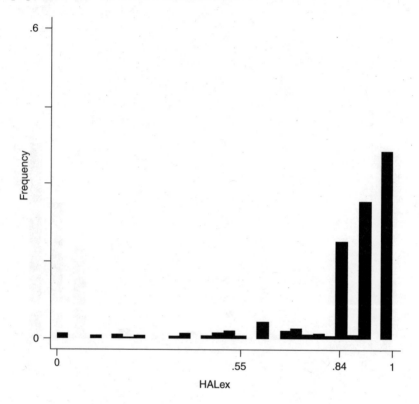

6 Did Health Equity Improve in the United States between 1990 and 1995?

6.1 Empirical Analyses from Different Perspectives on Health Equity

Using the tools developed in chapter 5, in this chapter I examine whether health equity improved in the United States between 1990 and 1995 from the following four different perspectives on health equity:[1]

- Health inequality as an indicator of social justice
- Health inequity as health inequality associated with a specific group characteristic
  - Race
  - Sex and gender
  - Education and income
- Health inequity as health inequality caused by socio-economic status
  - The Rawlsian Difference Principle
  - Walzer's view of dominance as unjust
- Health equity as satisfying the minimally adequate level of health (Capability Approach)

Health Inequality as an Indicator of Social Justice

First, I employ the view of health inequality as an indicator of social justice. Understanding health as an ultimate outcome of distributions of many important goods in our lives, in this perspective we perceive health inequality as carrying information on general social justice. From this perspective, did health equity improve in the United States between 1990 and 1995?

Let us recall figures 5.5 and 5.6, presented at the end of chapter 5.

Table 6.1
Health inequity analysis using the view of health inequality as an indicator of social justice: The Gini coefficient and variance of the HALex distribution for the living and the dead population in the United States in 1990 and 1995 by age and sex

	Both sexes		Male		Female	
	Gini	Variance	Gini	Variance	Gini	Variance
All ages						
1990	0.100	0.042	0.095	0.040	0.104	0.044
1995	0.104	0.044	0.099	0.042	0.108	0.046
0–14 years old						
1990	0.049	0.011	0.051	0.012	0.047	0.011
1995	0.050	0.012	0.053	0.013	0.047	0.010
15–24 years old						
1990	0.057	0.015	0.054	0.014	0.060	0.015
1995	0.061	0.016	0.058	0.015	0.064	0.017
25–44 years old						
1990	0.074	0.024	0.071	0.024	0.076	0.024
1995	0.081	0.028	0.078	0.027	0.083	0.028
45–64 years old						
1990	0.136	0.062	0.135	0.062	0.137	0.062
1995	0.138	0.062	0.137	0.064	0.139	0.061
65+ years old						
1990	0.218	0.115	0.214	0.115	0.220	0.115
1995	0.218	0.115	0.215	0.114	0.220	0.115

They illustrate how the HALex was distributed among the U.S. population of the living and the dead combined in 1990 and 1995, but it is obviously difficult to compare these figures as they are. Based on the discussion in chapters 4 and 5, I use the Gini coefficient as the health inequality measure with which the information in these figures can reasonably be summarized into one number. Tables 6.1 and 6.2 show the results. As a reference, results obtained by one of the simplest inequality measures, variance, are also listed.[2]

First, I look at the total U.S. population of the living and the dead combined (table 6.1). Between 1990 and 1995, the overall health inequality in the United States increased slightly (0.004 increase in the Gini coefficient). Health inequality among men and women had the same trend of the slight increase between these years (0.004 increase both for men and women). Every age group, except the elderly (65+ years old), observed this slight increase of health inequality between these years, with the largest increase among young adults (25–44 years old, 0.007 increase). Further stratifying by age group and sex, among men, health inequality increased in all age groups, while among women, health inequality increased among the adolescents (15–24 years old), young adults (25–44 years old), and adults (45–64 years old). From the perspective of health inequality as an indicator for general social justice, these results suggest that between 1990 and 1995, among the U.S. population of the living and the dead combined, general social justice slightly deteriorated, overall and among men and women, especially among young adults.

Next, I look at the living U.S. population (table 6.2). By excluding the dead, the Gini coefficients among the living population are smaller than those among the population of the living and the dead combined. Among the living, between 1990 and 1995, the overall health inequality increased slightly (0.005 increase in the Gini coefficient), and this increase is statistically significant at the 5% level. The same, statistically significant slight increase in health inequality was also observed among men (0.005 increase) and women (0.004 increase). Further stratifying the overall health inequality by sex and age group, it is clear that the source of health inequality of all ages comes from that of young adults (25–44 years old). Between 1990 and 1995, health inequality among young adults statistically significantly increased at the 5% level (0.007 increase). This was also true when young adults are stratified by sex (0.007 increase both for male and female young adults).

From the perspective of health inequality as an indicator of social justice, these results indicate that among the living U.S. population between 1990 and 1995, general social justice slightly but statistically significantly worsened at the 5% level, overall and both among men and women. And this general deterioration in social justice was led by the statistically significant worsening of general social justice among young adults (25–44 years old), both of men and women.

Health Inequity as Health Inequality Associated with a Specific Group Characteristic

In the section concerning the unit of analysis in chapter 3, I noted that people sometimes have a special interest in a specific group characteristic and define health inequity as health inequality associated with that group characteristic. Examples of such group characteristics include race, sex and gender, occupation, income, education, and

Table 6.2
The Gini coefficient and variance of the HALex distribution of the living population in the United States in 1990 and 1995 by age and sex

	Both sexes		Male		Female	
	Gini (95% CI)	Variance	Gini (95% CI)	Variance	Gini (95% CI)	Variance
All ages						
1990	0.092 (0.091, 0.094)	0.035	0.087 (0.086, 0.088)	0.032	0.097 (0.096, 0.099)	0.037
1995	0.097 (0.096, 0.099)	0.037	0.092 (0.090, 0.095)	0.035	0.101 (0.100, 0.103)	0.040
0–14 years old						
1990	0.048 (0.047, 0.049)	0.010	0.049 (0.048, 0.051)	0.011	0.046 (0.044, 0.048)	0.010
1995	0.049 (0.048, 0.050)	0.011	0.052 (0.050, 0.054)	0.012	0.046 (0.044, 0.048)	0.010
15–24 years old						
1990	0.056 (0.054, 0.059)	0.014	0.053 (0.050, 0.056)	0.013	0.059 (0.056, 0.062)	0.015
1995	0.060 (0.058, 0.062)	0.015	0.056 (0.053, 0.059)	0.014	0.063 (0.060, 0.066)	0.017
25–44 years old						
1990	0.072 (0.071, 0.074)	0.022	0.069 (0.067, 0.071)	0.022	0.075 (0.073, 0.077)	0.023
1995	0.079 (0.077, 0.081)	0.026	0.076 (0.074, 0.079)	0.025	0.082 (0.079, 0.084)	0.027
45–64 years old						
1990	0.127 (0.124, 0.130)	0.053	0.126 (0.122, 0.131)	0.054	0.127 (0.124, 0.131)	0.053
1995	0.132 (0.128, 0.138)	0.057	0.130 (0.123, 0.137)	0.056	0.134 (0.130, 0.140)	0.057
65+ years old						
1990	0.183 (0.178, 0.188)	0.084	0.172 (0.166, 0.178)	0.077	0.190 (0.184, 0.196)	0.089
1995	0.183 (0.174, 0.188)	0.084	0.174 (0.166, 0.183)	0.078	0.189 (0.177, 0.197)	0.088

geographic location. The perspective of health inequity as health inequality associated with a specific group characteristic is the most popular concept and the basis on which the vast majority of empirical analyses are conducted.

As I discussed in chapters 3 and 4, there are two problems with this popular approach to analysing health inequity. The first relates to the concept. When the concern brought by a specific group characteristic is legitimate for historical and political reasons, for example, race or ethnicity in the United States and South Africa, the health inequity analysis examining it may identify useful policy application. However, the question of which group characteristic causes inequitable health inequality is not usually carefully considered. Furthermore, health inequality associated with *any* group characteristic is often implied as inequitable.

The second problem of the popular approach is methodological. Customarily, health inequality by group is examined by comparing the average health between groups. But it is often questionable whose value is the average value, and as we saw in the section of the subpopulation decomposition of the Gini coefficient in chapter 5, a mere comparison of the average health between groups does not always reveal the extent of group stratification or isolation with respect to health.

In this section, I address these two problems by examining health inequality by such group characteristics as race, sex and gender, education, and income. As in other health inequity analyses using different perspectives on health equity, in the analyses in this section, I ask whether health inequity improved in the United States between 1990 and 1995. To do so, however, I first step back and examine what I mean by health inequity as health inequality associated with a group characteristic such as race, sex and gender, education, or income. After elaborating the concept, I measure health inequality by group by the decomposition technique introduced in chapter 5.

The group characteristics chosen for this section (that is, race, sex and gender, education, and income) are familiar ones for empirical analysis. Each analysis using each of these characteristics aims to show the two problems discussed above from different angles. The first analysis using race serves as an illustration of the effective use of the decomposition technique corresponding to the methodological problem discussed above. The second analysis using sex and gender warns the difficulty of using a seemingly straightforward variable, sex, in a conceptually sound way in health inequity analysis. The last analysis using education and income suggests that whether health inequality associated with education and income is inequitable depends on how one draws a line between individual free choice and social responsibility.

Due to the immaturity of the decomposition technique as a tool for health inequity analysis, age group stratification would complicate, rather than enrich, the analysis. In this section, therefore, I limit the analysis to all ages combined. Because age compositions of the U.S. populations in 1990 and 1995 are similar, the results will be comparable. In addition, in this section I only use the living population as I do not have the information on group characteristics for the dead imputed.[3]

RACE

Based on history and current social conditions, race in the United States is an important group characteristic for social justice considerations. It is not surprising that health inequality associated with race is considered to be inequitable.[4] With the first example of race, I therefore do not dispute the view that health inequality associated with race is inequitable. Rather, I use this example as an illustration of the effective use of the decomposition technique.

Table 6.3 summarizes the mean HALex and its 95% confidence intervals for White, Black, and other racial groups, differences in the mean HALex of these racial groups, the Gini coefficient and its 95% confidence intervals for these racial groups, and decomposition of the Gini coefficients by these racial groups. Did health equity improve in the United States between 1990 and 1995 from the perspective of health inequity as health inequality associated with race?

To answer this question, as explained in chapter 5, I propose to examine differences in the mean HALex of racial groups and contribution that the overlap term of the Gini coefficient makes to the overall Gini coefficient. Table 6.3 shows that the average HALex was lower in 1995 than 1990 in all three racial groups, although only the difference among Whites was statistically significant ($p<0.05$). Differences in the average HALex between all racial groups were the same in 1995 and 1990. Despite no difference in the average HALex between racial groups, the contribution of the overlap to the overall Gini coefficient was greater in 1995 than in 1990 by 2.3%. I therefore conclude that, from the perspective of health inequity as health inequality associated with race, health inequity improved in the United States between 1990 and 1995.[5] To tell how great this improvement was, we need further

Table 6.3

Health inequity analysis by race: The mean HALex, the Gini coefficient, and subgroup decomposition of the Gini coefficient for the living population in the United States in 1990 and 1995

	1990	1995
Mean HALex (95% CI)		
All	0.87 (0.87, 0.88)	0.87 (0.86, 0.87)
White	0.88 (0.88, 0.88)	0.87 (0.87, 0.87)
Black	0.85 (0.84, 0.85)	0.84 (0.84, 0.85)
Other	0.89 (0.88, 0.90)	0.88 (0.87, 0.89)
Mean HALex difference (* $p<0.05$)		
White – Black	0.03*	0.03*
Other – Black	0.04*	0.04*
Other – White	0.01	0.01
The Gini coefficient (95% CI)		
All	0.092 (0.091, 0.094)	0.097 (0.096, 0.099)
White	0.090 (0.089, 0.092)	0.095 (0.093, 0.098)
Black	0.109 (0.104, 0.115)	0.112 (0.109, 0.116)
Other	0.077 (0.072, 0.083)	0.085 (0.080, 0.092)
Decomposition of the Gini coefficient (Contribution, %)		
Overall	0.092 (100)	0.097 (100)
Between-group	0.004 (4.72)	0.004 (4.17)
Within-group	0.066 (71.47)	0.068 (69.69)
Overlap	0.022 (23.81)	0.025 (26.15)

methodological development of the use of the decomposition technique for health inequity analysis.

Let us now turn to unique information that the decomposition technique provides. Note that the contribution that the between-group Gini coefficient makes to the overall Gini coefficient is only 4.7% in 1990 and 4.2% in 1995. Literally interpreted, these numbers suggest that we would reduce only 4–5% of overall inequality even if the mean HALex of all three racial groups became magically the same. In addition, even when people shared a view of health inequity as health inequality associated with a specific group characteristic, race would hardly be the only group characteristic with which health inequity is defined. People would be interested in health inequity by, for example, gender, socioeconomic status, residence, or immigration status. Subgroup decomposition of the Gini coefficient would provide useful information when there are competing group characteristics; among health inequities identified as critical social problems, which one would contribute most to the overall health inequality?

While the decomposition technique provides unique information as discussed above, we must use it carefully. For example, regarding the small contribution that health inequality by race makes to overall health inequality, the importance of race for social justice consideration does not depend on the magnitude of the contribution that the between-group inequality makes to overall inequality. Even if there was a very small inequality in health by race, inequity is inequity: we ought to eliminate it. Moreover, which group characteristic would contribute most to the overall health inequality should not solely determine which group characteristic would be the best target for health equity policy. The overlap term at a point of time, for example, does not relate the historical persistence of health inequity by race in the United States.

SEX AND GENDER

Throughout part 1, I have emphasized two aspects of sex: sex as a biological determinant of health and sex as a social determinant of health, that is, gender. This distinction is important, I have argued, as to what makes a health distribution inequitable. We might not, for example, worry about men's generally shorter life span than women's if this were primarily determined by biology, for which no one can be responsible. We may, on the other hand, be concerned about higher incidence of violence among men than women if this related to the social expectation of how a man should be.

Unfortunately, in any empirical studies, sex and gender are not easily distinguishable. Using data from such a health interview survey as the NHIS, researchers only have information about the biological sex of a respondent. To judge that all observed health inequality by sex is inequitable implies that health inequality caused both by biological sex and gender is inequitable. In other words, if one treated all observed health inequality by sex as inequitable, one would be making an assumption about the variable, sex, that is, that both biological sex and gender cause inequitable health inequality. Such an assumption, unfortunately, is not often explicitly stated, or perhaps even recognized.

To examine whether health equity improved in the United States between 1990 and 1995 from the perspective of health inequity as health inequality by sex and gender, I take the position that health inequality associated with gender as well as biological sex is inequitable.

Table 6.4

Health inequity analysis by sex and gender: The mean HALex, the Gini coefficient, and subgroup decomposition of the Gini coefficient for the living population in the United States in 1990 and 1995

	1990	1995
Mean HALex (95% CI)		
Both sexes	0.87 (0.87, 0.88)	0.87 (0.86, 0.87)
Men	0.88 (0.88, 0.88)	0.87 (0.87, 0.88)
Women	0.87 (0.86, 0.87)	0.86 (0.86, 0.86)
Mean HALex difference (* p<0.05)		
Men – Women	0.01*	0.01*
The Gini coefficient (95% CI)		
Both sexes	0.092 (0.091, 0.094)	0.097 (0.096, 0.099)
Men	0.087 (0.086, 0.088)	0.092 (0.090, 0.095)
Women	0.097 (0.096, 0.099)	0.101 (0.100, 0.103)
Decomposition of the Gini coefficient (Contribution, %)		
Overall	0.092 (100)	0.097 (100)
Between-group	0.005 (5.23)	0.004 (4.58)
Within-group	0.046 (44.75)	0.048 (50.02)
Overlap	0.041 (50.03)	0.044 (45.40)

This position can be justified by the use of a health status measure, rather than life years, as the measurement of health.[6] It is much more uncertain whether biological sex makes any difference in a health-adjusted quality of life than in life years. And, even if it does, it is not clear whether we can easily dismiss such inequality as equitable. Obviously, further conceptual analysis is necessary on the issue of sex and gender. But I hope the discussion here is sufficient to warn that it is difficult to use a seemingly straightforward variable, sex, in a conceptually sound way.

As in the case of race, table 6.4 shows the mean HALex and its 95% confidence intervals for men and women in 1990 and 1995, differences in the mean HALex between men and women, the Gini coefficient and its 95% confidence intervals for men and women, and decomposition of the Gini coefficient by sex. Did health equity improve in the United States between 1990 and 1995 from the perspective of health inequity as health inequality associated with sex and gender? If we think that health inequality by gender and biological sex is inequitable, we can examine this question by

Table 6.5

Health inequity analysis by education as a proxy for socio-economic status: The mean HALex, the Gini coefficient, and subgroup decomposition of the Gini coefficient for the living population in the United States in 1990 and 1995

	1990	1995
Mean HALex (95% CI)		
All	0.84 (0.84, 0.85)	0.83 (0.83, 0.84)
Less than 12 years	0.73 (0.73, 0.74)	0.71 (0.71, 0.72)
12 years	0.85 (0.88, 0.88)	0.83 (0.83, 0.84)
13–15 years	0.88 (0.88, 0.88)	0.87 (0.86, 0.87)
16 years or more	0.91 (0.91, 0.91)	0.90 (0.90, 0.91)
Mean HALex difference (* $p<0.05$)		
(16+ years) – (Less than 12 years)	0.18*	0.19*
The Gini coefficient (95% CI)		
All	0.113 (0.112, 0.115)	0.118 (0.116, 0.122)
Less than 12 years	0.182 (0.178, 0.186)	0.194 (0.189, 0.200)
12 years	0.102 (0.099, 0.105)	0.113 (0.110, 0.116)
13–15 years	0.087 (0.084, 0.090)	0.094 (0.091, 0.099)
16 years or more	0.067 (0.065, 0.069)	0.069 (0.067, 0.073)
Decomposition of the Gini coefficient (Contribution, %)		
Overall	0.113 (100)	0.118 (100)
Between-group	0.038 (33.45)	0.040 (33.96)
Within-group	0.029 (25.55)	0.030 (25.06)
Overlap	0.046 (41.00)	0.048 (40.99)

looking at the differences in the mean HALex and the contribution that the overlap term makes to the overall Gini coefficient. The mean HALex difference was the same in 1990 and 1995, but the contribution that the overlap term makes to the overall Gini coefficient declined by 4.6% between 1990 and 1995. I thus conclude that health inequity deteriorated in the United States between 1990 and 1995 from the perspective of health inequity as health inequality associated with sex and gender.

EDUCATION AND INCOME

Education and income are other group characteristics whose relationships to health are often considered to cause moral concern. As discussed in chapters 2 and 3, they are often used as a proxy for socio-economic status (SES), following an intuitive belief that there is something unjust about unequal distribution of health by SES.[7] When income and education are used in this way, one would construct tables

Table 6.6
Health inequity analysis by income as a proxy for socio-economic status: The mean
HALex, the Gini coefficient, and subgroup decomposition of the Gini coefficient for the
living population in the United States in 1990 and 1995

	1990	1995
Mean HALex (95% CI)		
All	0.88 (0.88, 0.88)	0.87 (0.87, 0.87)
Less than $15,000	0.80 (0.79, 0.80)	0.79 (0.78, 0.79)
$15,000–$24,999	0.86 (0.85, 0.86)	0.83 (0.83, 0.84)
$25,000–$34,999	0.89 (0.90, 0.90)	0.88 (0.87, 0.88)
$35,000–$49,999	0.91 (0.91, 0.91)	0.90 (0.90, 0.90)
$50,000 or more	0.92 (0.92, 0.93)	0.92 (0.92, 0.92)
Mean HALex difference (* p<0.05) ($50,000 or more) – (Less than $15,000)	0.12*	0.13*
The Gini coefficient (95% CI)		
All	0.090 (0.089, 0.091)	0.095 (0.093, 0.097)
Less than $15,000	0.143 (0.140, 0.146)	0.152 (0.148, 0.157)
$15,000–$24,999	0.100 (0.096, 0.104)	0.117 (0.112, 0.122)
$25,000–$34,999	0.077 (0.073, 0.080)	0.086 (0.083, 0.089)
$35,000–$49,999	0.065 (0.062, 0.068)	0.071 (0.069, 0.074)
$50,000 or more	0.057 (0.055, 0.058)	0.057 (0.054, 0.059)
Decomposition of the Gini coefficient (Contribution, %)		
Overall	0.090 (100)	0.095 (100)
Between-group	0.028 (31.31)	0.031 (33.11)
Within-group	0.017 (19.27)	0.018 (19.05)
Overlap	0.045 (49.42)	0.045 (47.84)

6.5 and 6.6 for examining whether health equity improved in the
United States between 1990 and 1995.

Table 6.5 facilitates the analysis when education is used as a proxy for
SES. The difference in the mean HALex between the top and bottom
education groups was greater in 1995 than in 1990 by 0.01, while the
overlap stayed almost the same between these years. I thus conclude
that from the perspective of health inequity as health inequality associated with education (as a proxy for SES), health equity in the United
States deteriorated between 1990 and 1995.

Similarly, for the case of using income as a proxy for SES, one would
look at table 6.6 to examine health equity by income in the United
States between 1990 and 1995 (see appendix F for the issue of adjust-

ment of household income for the family size and structure). The difference in the mean HALex between the top and bottom income groups increased by 0.01 between 1990 and 1995, and the contribution that the overlap term makes to the Gini coefficient decreased by 1.6% in this period. Thus, from the perspective of health inequity as health inequality associated with income (as a proxy for SES), health equity in the United States deteriorated between 1990 and 1995.

Despite the extensive use of income and education as a proxy for SES, it is no surprise that some people are uncomfortable with such application. Using income and education as a proxy for SES assumes that they reflect the basic social structure, in other words, their distributions are primarily determined by social arrangement rather than individual choice. Throughout this book, I have emphasized the difficulty in drawing a line between individual free choice and social responsibility (for example, see section 2.2 in chapter 2). Various socio-economic factors no doubt influence one's educational path and income earnings, but individuals do make, at least to some degree, their own decisions about how much education to obtain and how much money to earn. If one were serious about granting an individual choice, then, one could not make the assumption that distributions of education and income are largely socially determined. In this case, education and income cannot be used as a proxy for SES, and one would not consider health inequality across all education or income groups as inequitable.

What, then, is inequitable? Recall that inequity suggests a social responsibility. Inequitable health inequality calls upon social consideration and action. The question is therefore better rephrased: granting individual choice on educational attainment and income earnings, which part of health inequality associated with income or education ought society to be concerned about?

In the case of education, one may only be concerned about how much difference to health a compulsory education can make. For a variety of reasons, it is widely known that the higher a person's educational attainment is, the healthier she is. To the extent that the choice to pursue higher education is personal, the additional health benefit attached to a higher education is also a personal choice. Society, then, would not need to be responsible for the health of those who make a decision to pursue higher education. What society should be concerned about is how much health can be produced by compulsory education, that is, a social responsibility.

If this was the view, the measurement strategy would accordingly need to be altered from the previous analysis. The right focus would be to see how those who have twelve years or less of education fare in terms of health in 1990 and 1995. Table 6.5 shows that the mean HALex of these two groups decreased by 0.02 HALex in 1995 from 1990. The reduction in both groups was statistically significant at the 5% level. The Gini coefficient increased statistically significantly at the 5% level during these years (0.012 increase for people with fewer than twelve years of education, and 0.011 increase for people with twelve years of education). As an overall conclusion, from the perspective of health inequity as health inequality associated with education (and under the assumption that individuals do make decisions on educational attainment and a society should be responsible only for the health of those who have, or have less than, compulsory education), health equity in the United States deteriorated between 1990 and 1995.

In the case of income, similar to the cut-off point of compulsory education, one might think that a society should be responsible for the health of those who are below the poverty line. It is now common knowledge that the higher somebody's income is, the healthier that person is. As for the case of education, if people make a decision on how much money they want to earn, then, the better health that comes with a higher income is also their choice. In this view, society would not worry about the health of people with higher incomes. What level of income is considered as a personal choice is a point of dispute, but as society has decided to help people below the poverty line, it can also be concerned about their health.

Table 6.7 shows the mean HALex, the Gini coefficient, and their 95% confidence intervals for those who below the poverty line in 1990 and 1995. The mean HALex of those below the poverty line declined from 0.82 to 0.81 between 1990 and 1995, and this 0.01 reduction is statistically significant at the 5% level. Furthermore, between these years, the Gini coefficient of the HALex among people below the poverty line increased by a statistically significant 0.011 at the 5% level. Based on this result, from the perspective of health inequity as health inequality associated with income (and under the assumption that individuals make decisions on their income earning), health equity in the United States deteriorated between 1990 and 1995.

Health Inequity as Health Inequality Caused by Socio-economic Status

THE RAWLSIAN DIFFERENCE PRINCIPLE

In chapter 3, I introduced John Rawls's theory of justice as fairness (1971) as a possible philosophical theory to explain why health inequal-

Table 6.7

Health inequity analysis by income (choice granted): The mean HALex and the Gini coefficient for the living population in the United States in 1990 and 1995

	1990	1995
Mean HALex (95% CI)		
All	0.88 (0.88, 0.88)	0.87 (0.87, 0.87)
Below the poverty line	0.82 (0.82, 0.83)	0.81 (0.80, 0.81)
At or above the poverty line	0.89 (0.88, 0.89)	0.88 (0.88, 0.88)
The Gini coefficient (95% CI)		
All	0.089 (0.088, 0.090)	0.094 (0.092, 0.096)
Below the poverty line	0.126 (0.122, 0.130)	0.137 (0.134, 0.141)
At or above the poverty line	0.084 (0.082, 0.085)	0.087 (0.085, 0.089)

ity caused by socio-economic status (SES) might be inequitable. Rawls does not consider health as a social primary good whose distribution causes concern for justice in his theory. Various proposals have been suggested to incorporate health into the Rawlsian framework, and one such proposal is to include health in the list of social primary goods and consider it as a good governed by the difference principle. The difference principle directs that inequality is permissible only if redistribution improves the position of the worst-off. The inclusion of health in the social primary goods complicates indexing the holding of the entire social primary goods. Rawls suggests income as the index, but when health is included, it is not clear what makes the best index.

Although numerous issues need to be solved before Rawls's theory of justice as fairness can be used as a solid foundation for health inequity analysis, below I assume all of these issues are solved. Specifically, I assume that health can be included in the list of social primary goods, that health can be governed by the difference principle, and that the index of the holding of the social primary goods is still income. Under these assumptions, using Rawls's difference principle, did health equity improve in the United States between 1990 and 1995?

The worst-off group, indexed by income, is the bottom income group of family income less than $15,000 in table 6.6.[8] Table 6.8 shows that the mean HALex of the bottom income group for all ages did not change statistically significantly between 1990 and 1995. During these years, the Gini coefficient of the HALex in the bottom income group for all ages increased from 0.143 to 0.152, and the 0.009 increase is statistically

Table 6.8
Health inequity analysis using the Rawlsian difference principle: The mean HALex and the Gini coefficient of the bottom income group (less than $15,000) for the living population in the United States in 1990 and 1995 by age

	Mean HALex (95% CI)	Gini coefficient (95% CI)
All ages		
1990	0.80 (0.79, 0.80)	0.143 (0.140, 0.146)
1995	0.79 (0.78, 0.79)	0.152 (0.148, 0.157)
0–14 years old		
1990	0.90 (0.90, 0.91)	0.063 (0.059, 0.067)
1995	0.90 (0.89, 0.90)	0.067 (0.064, 0.071)
15–24 years old		
1990	0.89 (0.89, 0.90)	0.071 (0.066, 0.075)
1995	0.88 (0.88, 0.89)	0.075 (0.068, 0.080)
25–44 years old		
1990	0.82 (0.81, 0.83)	0.125 (0.118, 0.131)
1995	0.79 (0.78, 0.79)	0.147 (0.138, 0.155)
45–64 years old		
1990	0.65 (0.64, 0.66)	0.238 (0.229, 0.246)
1995	0.62 (0.61, 0.64)	0.252 (0.243, 0.263)
65+ years old		
1990	0.68 (0.67, 0.69)	0.210 (0.200, 0.219)
1995	0.67 (0.66, 0.68)	0.217 (0.204, 0.227)

significant at the 5% level. These results suggest that, overall, the bottom income group in 1990 and 1995 fared the same in terms of health equity, while the bottom income group in 1995 fared worse than that of 1995 when examining health distribution within the group. I thus conclude that from the perspective of health inequity as health inequality caused by SES in adoption of the difference principle, health equity in the United States deteriorated between 1990 and 1995.

Table 6.8 also shows the mean HALex and its Gini coefficient of the bottom income group by age group. Note that no statistically significant change was observed in the mean HALex and the Gini coefficient between 1990 and 1995 among children (0–14 years old), adolescents (15–24 years old), adults (45–64 years old) and the elderly (65+ years old). Among young adults (25–44 years old), the mean HALex decreased by 0.03, and the Gini coefficient increased by 0.022. Both of these changes are statistically significant at the 5% level. To summarize, from the perspective on health equity using the difference principle, between 1990 and 1995 health equity in the United States deteriorated among young adults.

WALZER'S VIEW OF DOMINANCE AS UNJUST
Chapter 3 introduced Walzer's complex inequality (1983) as another philosophical theory that might give a solid conceptual foundation for why health inequality caused by socio-economic status (SES) is inequitable. Walzer thinks that there are various independent spheres of justice, each of them governed by different rules. What should concern us as inequitable, Walzer argues, is not inequality within each sphere, but the concentration of burdens and prestige. Applying this view of dominance as unjust to health, health inequality itself does not cause moral concern, but its correlations with other spheres do.

When applying Walzer's view, one must define what spheres of justice are. Here I make a provisional simplification: income and education. Health distribution is inequitable when the rich and the educated are healthy while the poor and the uneducated are sick. From this perspective, we are interested in correlations between health and education, and health and income. These correlations can be examined by decomposing the Gini coefficient by educational or income groups, and looking at the overlap term. A greater overlap indicates more difficulty to predict the health level of a person by educational attainment or income earnings. Thus, a greater overlap is a sign of equity in Walzer's view of dominance as unjust. Using Walzer's view of dominance as unjust, did health equity improve in the United States between 1990 and 1995?[9]

Table 6.9 presents the decomposition of the Gini coefficient by education and income groups in 1990 and 1995. Categorizations of education and income are the same as in previous analyses. For education, contribution of the overlap term for the overall Gini coefficient stayed almost the same between 1990 and 1995 (−0.01% reduction). For income, it reduced slightly, 1.6%, during these years. These overlap terms together suggest that, from the perspective of health inequity as health inequality caused by SES, applying Walzer's view of dominance as unjust, health equity slightly deteriorated in the United States between 1990 and 1995.

Health Equity as Satisfying the Minimally Adequate Level of Health (Capability Approach)

The last empirical analysis in this chapter adopts the view of health equity as satisfying the minimally adequate level of health. Specifically,

Table 6.9
Health inequity analysis using Walzer's view of dominance as unjust: Subgroup
decomposition of the Gini coefficient (contribution, %) by education and income
for the living population in the United States in 1990 and 1995

	1990	1995
By education		
Overall	0.113 (100)	0.118 (100)
Between-group	0.038 (33.45)	0.040 (33.96)
Within-group	0.029 (25.55)	0.030 (25.06)
Overlap	0.046 (41.00)	0.048 (40.99)
By income		
Overall	0.090 (100)	0.095 (100)
Between-group	0.028 (31.31)	0.031 (33.11)
Within-group	0.017 (19.27)	0.018 (19.05)
Overlap	0.045 (49.42)	0.045 (47.84)

I use Nussbaum's version of the capability approach (2000). I define the minimally adequate level of health as the average level of health in each age and sex group. In other words, in the following analysis the minimally adequate level of health changes from 1990 to 1995, for men and women, and for different age groups. This definition is arbitrary, but it makes sense if the average level of health in each age and sex is thought of as the health that society can reasonably offer to its members. Change in the minimally adequate level of health by study year reflects general resources available for health development around study years in a given society, and stratification by sex and age group takes biological effects on health into considerations.[10] Based on the discussion in the section above of the measurement of health equity, I use the Foster-Greer-Thorbecke (FGT) measure ($\alpha = 2$) (Foster, Greer, and Thorbecke 1984) as the measurement of health inequity. As I explained in section 5.2, α in the FGT measure expresses the sensitivity to the health gap, that is, how far off the sick are from the threshold. A larger α assigns a greater weight to the sick below the threshold, and the FGT measure is the head-count ratio when $\alpha = 0$, the health-gap index when =1, and the squared health-gap index when $\alpha = 2$. To help interpret results, the FGT measure ($\alpha = 0$) and ($\alpha = 1$) will also be presented along with the FGT measure ($\alpha = 2$).

In chapter 3, I discussed a number of difficulties that the idea of the minimally adequate level of health presents. As with other perspectives on health equity, this view is not flawless. Nevertheless, again I assume

Table 6.10
Health inequity analysis using the capability approach: Health inequity measured by
the FGT measures for the living and dead population in the United States in 1990 and
1995 by age

	Threshold health (HALex)[a]	Degree of health inequity[b]	Individuals below threshold (%)[c]	Average lack of health over the whole population (HALex)[d]
All ages				
1990	0.87	0.031	34.9	0.06
1995	0.86	0.033	36.6	0.06
0–14 years old				
1990	0.93	0.008	48.2	0.03
1995	0.93	0.009	48.3	0.04
15–24 years old				
1990	0.92	0.011	26.2	0.04
1995	0.91	0.013	27.7	0.04
25–44 years old				
1990	0.90	0.019	30.5	0.05
1995	0.90	0.24	33.2	0.06
45–64 years old				
1990	0.81	0.047	26.1	0.08
1995	0.81	0.051	26.5	0.08
65+ years old				
1990	0.70	0.071	33.1	0.09
1995	0.70	0.071	33.5	0.09

[a] The average level of health in each category
[b] Based on FGT ($\alpha = 2$)
[c] Based on FGT ($\alpha = 0$, the head-count index) x 100
[d] Based on FGT ($\alpha = 1$, the gap index) x threshold health

that all problems have been solved and the idea of the minimally adequate level of health can provide a strong basis for health inequity analysis. With these assumptions, from the perspective of health equity as
satisfying the minimally adequate level of health, did health equity
improve in the United States between 1990 and 1995?

Table 6.10 shows results for the U.S. population of the living and the
dead combined in 1990 and 1995 by age group. Table 6.11 presents
results for the U.S. living population in 1990 and 1995 by age group.
The threshold health is, as mentioned above, the average HALex in
each category. The degree of health inequity is calculated by the FGT

measure ($\alpha = 2$). The calculation of the proportion of individuals below the threshold is based on the FGT measure ($\alpha = 0$). The average lack of health measured in the HALex over the whole population is derived from the FGT measure ($\alpha = 1$). In addition to these numbers, table 6.11 also presents 95% confidence intervals for the degree of health inequity.

Let us first look at the total population of the living and the dead combined. Table 6.10 shows that overall health inequity slightly deteriorated (0.002 increase in the FGT measure [$\alpha = 2$]) between 1990 and 1995. This is also apparent in the slight increase in individuals below the minimally adequate level of health (1.7% increase). Both men and women provided the same picture (0.002 increase in the FGT measure [$\alpha = 2$] for men, and 0.002 increase for women, data not shown).

Table 6.10 also suggests that health inequity worsened between 1990 and 1995 in every age group, except among the elderly (65+ years old), with the worst deterioration observed among young adults (25–44 years old, 0.005 increase in the FGT measure [$\alpha = 2$]). Among men, health inequity deteriorated in every age group, while among women the deterioration is observed only among the adolescent (15–24 years old), young adults (25–44 years old), and adults (45–64 years old) (data not shown). From the perspective of health equality as satisfying the minimally adequate level of health, these results suggest that between 1990 and 1995, among the U.S. population of the living and the dead combined, health equity deteriorated slightly, both overall and among men and women, especially among young adults (25–44 years old) and adults (45–64 years old).

Next, let us look at the living population (table 6.11). First note that the exclusion of the dead does not necessarily result in improvement in health equity, as in the case of analysis using the Gini coefficient. This is because the minimally adequate level of health is different in the total population, including the dead and the living population only. Table 6.11 shows that between 1990 and 1995 overall health equity did not change statistically significantly among the living U.S. population at the 5% level. Between these years, individuals below the threshold increased by 1.0% but the average lack of the HALex over the whole population was the same. Both men and women did not have statistically significant change (data not shown).

Confidence intervals suggest that between 1990 and 1995 health equity worsened statistically significantly at the 5% level only among young adults (25–44 years old). There was a decline of 0.004 in the FGT

Table 6.11

Health inequity analysis using the capability approach: Health inequity measured by the FGT measures for the living population in the United States in 1990 and 1995 by age

	Threshold health (HALex)[a]	Degree of health inequity[b]	Individuals below threshold (%)[c]	Average lack of health over the whole population (HALex)[d]
All ages				
1990	0.87	0.031 (0.030, 0.032)	35.6	0.06
1995	0.87	0.033 (0.032, 0.035)	36.6	0.06
0–14 years old				
1990	0.93	0.008 (0.008, 0.009)	48.2	0.03
1995	0.93	0.009 (0.008, 0.010)	48.3	0.04
15–24 years old				
1990	0.92	0.011 (0.011, 0.012)	26.2	0.04
1995	0.91	0.013 (0.012, 0.014)	27.7	0.04
25–44 years old				
1990	0.90	0.019 (0.018, 0.020)	30.5	0.05
1995	0.89	0.023 (0.022, 0.024)	33.2	0.05
45–64 years old				
1990	0.82	0.048 (0.046, 0.050)	26.1	0.08
1995	0.81	0.052 (0.049, 0.054)	27.1	0.08
65+ years old				
1990	0.73	0.077 (0.073, 0.080)	40.7	0.10
1995	0.73	0.077 (0.074, 0.080)	41.6	0.10

[a] The average level of health in each category
[b] Based on FGT ($\alpha = 2$)
[c] Based on FGT ($\alpha = 0$, the head-count index) x 100
[d] Based on FGT ($\alpha = 1$, the gap index) x threshold health

measure ($\alpha = 2$), and 2.7% more people were below the threshold in 1995 than 1990, although the average lack of the HALex over the whole population between these years was the same, 0.05. Further stratifying by sex, only women aged 25–44 years old had the same result of statistically significant deterioration of health equity (0.004 increase, data not shown). Therefore, from the perspective of health equity as satisfying the minimally adequate level of health, health equity among the living population in the United States did not change statistically significantly at the 5% level between 1990 and 1995, and but among young adults (25–44 years old) health equity deteriorated.

Previously I discussed the potential of the decomposition of the FGT measure by subpopulation for health equity policy-making. Now let us discuss further this potential with an example. In chapter 3 (section 3.5), I concluded that the idea of the minimally adequate level of health was the only perspective on health equity discussed in this project to strongly favour the individual as the unit of analysis. Hence, the health inequity analysis above, using the individual as the unit of analysis, is sound, but it is difficult to use the results for policy-making. In the attempt to improve observed health inequity, it will be useful to know which group – in addition to groups defined by health status – is possibly a good target for effective improvement. Decomposition of the FGT measure is a helpful tool for such identification. As an example, let us ask: which group is the best target if we wish to improve health equity among young adults (25–44 years old)?

Table 6.12 shows results of the decomposition of the FGT measure ($\alpha = 2$) by race, education, income, and poverty for young adults in 1995. The third column of the 'contribution to total inequity' is the key in these results. Let us look at the decomposition results for Whites and Blacks. Health inequity among Blacks is statistically significantly worse than among Whites by 0.016 in the FGT measure ($\alpha = 2$) at the 5% level. How many people were below the threshold among Whites and Blacks, and on average, how far off were they from the threshold? Among Blacks, 12.1% more people are below the threshold than among Whites, and Black people below the threshold lack 0.03 more HALex on average than White people below the threshold. Despite the fact that health inequity is much worse among Blacks than Whites, from the column of the 'contribution to total inequity' we learn that Whites' contribution to total inequality is 76.5% and Blacks' 19.6%. This means that if we could somehow successfully bring all Whites to or above the minimally adequate level of health, 76.5% of the total health inequity currently observed will disappear, while for the case of Blacks, the effect is a 19.6% reduction. Recall that additively decomposable poverty measures use population share as a weight for decomposition.[11] This is why the contribution of Whites is much greater than that of Blacks despite Blacks having worse health inequity than Whites.

To decide which group is the best target to improve health equity, we should not only be concerned about which group would bring the greatest expected change. As I discussed in the analysis using the view of health inequity as health inequality by race, we must take into account many other considerations. For example, we might place a

Table 6.12
Subpopulation decomposition of the FGT measures for the living population of 25–44 years old in the United States in 1995

	Population share (%)	Degree of health inequity (95% CI)[a]	Contribution to total inequity (%)	Average health of individuals below threshold (HALex)	Individuals below threshold (%)[b]	Average lack of health over the whole population (HALex)[c]
Race						
White	82.7	0.021 (0.020, 0.023)	76.5	0.73	31.5	0.05
Black	12.3	0.037 (0.033, 0.041)	19.6	0.71	43.6	0.08
Other	5.1	0.018 (0.014, 0.022)	3.9	0.76	35.7	0.04
Total	100	0.023 (0.022, 0.024)	100	0.73	33.2	0.05
Education						
Less than 12 years	12.2	0.058 (0.053, 0.062)	30.5	0.69	56.4	0.11
12 years	36.8	0.025 (0.023, 0.026)	39.7	0.73	37.7	0.06
13–15 years	24.1	0.019 (0.017, 0.021)	20.3	0.73	29.1	0.04
16 years or more	26.9	0.008 (0.007, 0.009)	9.5	0.77	19.9	0.02
Total	100	0.023 (0.022, 0.024)	100	0.73	33.1	0.05
Income						
Less than $15,000	13.2	0.071 (0.066, 0.077)	41.1	0.65	55.9	0.06
$15,000–$24,999	16.1	0.031 (0.028, 0.034)	21.7	0.72	41.8	0.03
$25,000–$34,999	17.5	0.018 (0.015, 0.020)	13.5	0.75	32.6	0.02
$35,000–$49,999	22.2	0.013 (0.011, 0.014)	12.4	0.76	28.2	0.01
$50,000 or more	31.0	0.008 (0.007, 0.009)	11.3	0.77	21.4	0.01
Total	100	0.023 (0.022, 0.024)	100	0.73	32.7	0.05
Poverty						
Below	9.8	0.072 (0.065, 0.078)	31.9	0.66	59.5	0.14
At or above	90.2	0.017 (0.016, 0.018)	68.1	0.75	29.4	0.04
Total	100	0.022 (0.021, 0.023)	100	0.73	32.4	0.05

[a] Based on FGT ($\alpha = 2$)
[b] Based on FGT ($\alpha = 0$, the head-count index) x 100
[c] Based on FGT ($\alpha = 1$, the gap index) x threshold health
The minimally adequate level of health (threshold) measured by the HALex=0.89

priority on a specific subgroup for reasons unrelated to health equity considerations. Even within health equity considerations, which group would benefit most is but one consideration, and, for example, historical persistence of inequitable treatment of a specific group does not appear in data we have here. Still, I believe the contribution to total inequity is a useful figure. In addition, from various options of group characteristics and categorization of a chosen group characteristic, the decomposition technique can serve as a simulation tool for a proposal for improving health equity.

Table 6.13 summarizes definitions of health equity used in health inequity analyses in part 2, and table 6.14 results of analyses in part 2. Given the limited space, for the total population of the living and the dead combined, only overall results, that is, all ages and both sexes, are presented in table 6.14.

6.2 Discussion

Health Equity in the United States Deteriorated between 1990 and 1995

Whichever the perspective on health equity used for analysis, table 6.14 shows that health equity in the United States deteriorated between 1990 and 1995 in most cases. Moreover, age group analysis in the view of health inequality as an indicator of social justice, the Rawlsian difference principle, and the view of health equity as satisfying the minimally adequate level of health all suggest that the deterioration is primarily due to that of young adults (25–44 years old). This points to the need for targeting young adults in health equity policy-making irrespective of the exact conception of health equity employed. This result also requires further investigation of 'sensitivity analysis' of different perspectives on health equity in the actual application in empirical studies. At the conceptual level, different equity perspectives have distinct characteristics, but how many of these characteristics actually carry over to empirical investigation?

Why Did Health Equity in the United States Worsen between 1990 and 1995? Comparison to Japan

Given the fairly uniform results of deteriorating health equity in the United States, a question that naturally comes to mind is possible reasons why this happened. The analyses in part 2 are not designed to

Table 6.13
Summary of definitions of health equity used in analyses in part 2

Health equity perspective	Which health distribution is inequitable?
Health inequality as an indicator of social justice	All health inequalities are considered as carrying information on general social justice
Health inequity as health inequality associated with:	
Race	Difference in the average levels of health between racial groups and stratification of health by racial group
Sex/gender	Difference in the average levels of health between men and women and stratification of health by sex and gender
Education (as a proxy for SES)	Difference in the average levels of health between education groups and stratification of health by education group
Education (choice granted)	Reduction of the average level of health of those who have a compulsory education or less and not higher
Income (as a proxy for SES)	Difference in the average levels of health between income groups and stratification of health by income group
Income (choice granted)	Reduction of the average level of health of those who are below the poverty line
Health inequity as health inequality associated with socio-economic status:	
The Rawlsian difference principle	Reduction of the average level of health of the worst-off (the lowest income level)
Walzer's view of dominance as unjust	Stratification of health by income and education
Health equity as satisfying the minimally adequate level of health	Shortfalls of health from the minimally adequate level of health (the average health of a group stratified by sex and age group)

identify such reasons, but I can speculate about them. To do so, a comparison to a similar study is useful, and here I take an example of the analysis of health inequity in Japan from the perspective of health inequality as an indicator of social justice.[12]

In this analysis, my colleague and I used a Japanese national health survey, the Comprehensive Survey of Living Conditions of the People on Health and Welfare conducted by the Japanese Ministry of Health, Labour and Welfare. This is a cross-sectional survey, and we used 1989 and 1998 data. With modification, we applied the HALex to this data set and conducted a parallel analysis to the one in this chapter with the view of health inequality as an indicator of social justice. Cross-cultural application of the HALex remains an issue, and data years are not exactly comparable. Nonetheless, it is insightful to see the U.S. and Japanese results side by side.

Table 6.15 compares changes in life expectancy, the average HALex, and inequality in the HALex (of the living population) measured by the Gini coefficient in the United States and Japan in the 1990s. In both countries, in the 1990s women were expected to live longer than men, but women's HALex was on average lower than men's. In both countries, during the 1990s life expectancies improved but the average HALex stayed about the same for both men and women. Inequality in the HALex, however, increased during the 1990s in the United States both for men and women, while inequality in the HALex stayed about the same during the 1990s in Japan both for men and women. This means that, understanding health inequality as an indicator of general social justice, during the 1990s American society worsened but Japanese society stayed about the same in terms of social justice. What happened, or did not happen, in the United States in the 1990s?

One obvious object of speculation is the relationship between health and income. In early 1990s, the United States experienced major economic growth that benefited the wealthy rather than the poor.[13] An increase in income inequality, rather than general economic growth, might have had a greater effect on population health production. If this was a plausible hypothesis, future analysis must be more sensitive to income and poverty variables than my analyses were. I did not, for example, adjust for inflation between 1990 and 1995, and I used a rough categorization of income groups. Future studies may need to be more careful about the construction of income and poverty variables.

The 'Forgotten' Age Group (25–44 years old)

It is surprising to find that health equity among young adults (25–44 years old) deteriorated between 1990 and 1995. A possible etiology for this deterioration is the spread of HIV/AIDS (human immunodeficiency virus/acquired immunodeficiency syndrome); in 1995, HIV/AIDS was the leading cause of death among young adults (Anderson, Kochanek,

Table 6.14
Summary of results of analyses in part 2

Health equity perspective	Target population	Between 1990 and 1995, health equity...	Magnitude
Health inequality as an indicator of social justice	The living + the dead, overall	deteriorated	+ 0.004 in Gini
	The living, overall	deteriorated	+ 0.005 in Gini[a]
	The living, men	deteriorated	+ 0.005 in Gini[a]
	The living, women	deteriorated	+ 0.004 in Gini[a]
	The living, 25–44 years old	deteriorated	+ 0.007 in Gini[a]
	The living, other age groups	did not change statistically significantly	
Health inequity as health inequality associated with			
Race	The living, overall	improved	+ 2.3% in overlap Gini
Sex and gender	The living, overall	deteriorated	– 4.6% in overlap Gini
Education (as a proxy for SES)	The living, overall	deteriorated	+ 0.01 in difference in HALex[b]
Education (choice granted)	The living, overall	deteriorated	– 0.02 in HALex for <12 yr education[a]
			+ 0.012 in Gini for <12 yr education[a]
			– 0.02 in HALex for 12 yr education[a]
			+ 0.011 in Gini for 12 yr education[a]
Income (as a proxy for SES)	The living, overall	deteriorated	+ 0.01 in difference in HALex[c]
			– 1.6% overlap Gini
Income (choice granted)	The living, overall	deteriorated	– 0.01 in HALex for below poverty line[a]
			+ 0.011 in Gini for below poverty line[a]

Table 6.14 — (continued)

Health equity perspective	Target population	Between 1990 and 1995, health equity...	Magnitude
Rawlsian Difference Principle	The living, overall	deteriorated	+ 0.009 in Gini for <$15,000 income[a]
	The living, 25–44 years old	deteriorated	− 0.03 in HALex for <$15,000 income[a]
			+ 0.022 in Gini for <$15,000 income[a]
	The living, other age groups	did not change statistically significantly	
Walzer's view of dominance as unjust	The living, overall	deteriorated	− 0.01% in overlap Gini for education
			− 1.6% in overlap Gini for income
Health equity as satisfying the minimally adequate level of health	The living + the dead, overall	deteriorated	+ 0.002 in FGT
	The living, overall	did not change statistically significantly	
	The living, men	did not change statistically significantly	
	The living, women	did not change statistically significantly	
	The living, 25–44 years old	deteriorated	+ 0.004 in FGT[a]
	The living, other age groups	did not change statistically significantly	

a Statistically significant change (5%)
b Top education group (16 years or more) – bottom education group (less than 12 years)
c Top income group ($50,000 or more) – bottom income group (less than $15,000)

Table 6.15

Life expectancy, the average HALex, and inequality in the HALex in the United States and Japan around 1990 and in the mid-1990s by sex

	United States		Japan	
	Male	Female	Male	Female
Life expectancy, year				
Around 1990[a]	71.8	78.8	75.2	81.8
Mid-1990s[b]	72.5	78.9	77.2	84.0
Change	+ 0.7	+ 0.1	+ 2.0	+ 2.2
Average HALex				
Around 1990	0.88	0.87	0.87	0.85
Mid-1990s	0.87	0.86	0.86	0.84
Change	−0.01	−0.01	−0.01	−0.01
Inequality in the HALex[c]				
Around 1990	0.087	0.097	0.085	0.095
Mid-1990s	0.092	0.101	0.086	0.096
Change	+ 0.005	+ 0.004	+ 0.001	+ 0.001

[a] 1990 for the United States, 1989 for Japan
[b] 1995 for the United States, 1998 for Japan
[c] Measured by the Gini coefficient

and Murphy 1997). Nonetheless, even without the prevalence of HIV/AIDS, this might still be called the 'forgotten' age group. Health policy tends to focus on infants, adolescents, and the elderly. Young adulthood is often considered the most resilient stage of life in terms of human biology. It is, however, this period of life in which the proportion of the uninsured is the second highest (after 18–24 years old) (Families USA 2003), and many people struggle to establish themselves as young families. To investigate why health equity among young adults in particular deteriorated between 1990 and 1995, it might be interesting to examine how the economic growth in early 1990s affected the health production and health care of this age group. Methodologically, decomposing health inequity in a multivariate fashion would be useful to investigate reasons for the worsening health equity among young adults.

Health Inequality Associated with Race

Among the bad news of worsening health equity in the United States, a notable exception is the view of health inequity as health inequality associated with race: from this perspective, health equity improved between

1990 and 1995. This observation of the improvement in health equity between racial or ethnic groups in the early 1990s is compatible with findings of other studies. In 1990, for example, life expectancy was 69.1 years for Blacks and 76.1 years for Whites (National Center for Health Statistics 1994), and in 1995, 69.6 years for Blacks and 76.5 years for Whites (National Center for Health Statistics 1998). Between these years, life expectancy both for Blacks and Whites improved (0.5 year improvement for Blacks and 0.4 year improvement for Whites), and the difference in life expectancy between Blacks and Whites declined slightly (0.1 year) due to the marginally better improvement among Blacks than Whites.

As a follow-up to *Healthy People 2000*, Keppel, Pearcy, and Wagener examined differences in all-cause mortality rates by race/ethnicity between 1990 and 1998 (Keppel, Pearcy, and Wagener 2002; Pearcy and Keppel 2002). They used five racial or ethnic groups: non-Hispanic White, non-Hispanic Black, Hispanic, American Indian or Alaska Native, and Asian or Pacific Islander. Between 1990 and 1998, all racial or ethnic groups, except American Indian or Alaska Native, reduced all-cause mortality rates. The index of disparity, the measure of health inequality used in this study, indicated that between 1990 and 1998 the difference in all-cause mortality by race/ethnicity statistically significantly reduced by 7.2% at the 5% level.[14] These two observations and the analysis in part 2 suggest that, whether looking at life years or health-adjusted quality of life, from the view of health inequity as health inequality associated with race or ethnicity, health equity improved between 1990 and 1995. A caution for this welcome finding is that the improvement in health equity in terms of the HALex came in the general trend of no change in the HALex between 1990 and 1995, while the improvement in health equity in terms of life years occurred with increasing life years to almost all racial or ethnic groups between these years.

The categorization of racial groups is a major limitation of this study. The 'other' group limits further meaningful comparisons of this study to other studies. Given that this study showed the average HALex was highest and its inequality was lowest in the 'other' racial group both in 1990 and 1995, the further classification of this group would provide useful information on the health of different racial groups in the United States.

Recommendations for Healthy People 2010

Analyses using the view of health inequity as health inequality associated with race and other group characteristics and Walzer's view of dominance as unjust show the potential of the decomposition technique in health equity analysis. Application of the subpopulation decomposition technique to health inequity analysis is still in its infancy, and this has led to ambiguity of some results.

Despite the ambiguity, my analyses using the view of health inequity as health inequality associated with specific group characteristics give a caution to the widespread assumption that health inequality associated with *any* group characteristic is inequitable. As quoted already in previous chapters, the second goal of *Healthy People 2010* is 'to eliminate health disparities among segments of the population, including differences that occur by gender, race or ethnicity, education or income, disability, geographic location, or sexual orientation' (U.S. Department of Health and Human Services 2000). For this to be a sound goal, we must first look at the conceptual validity of perceiving health inequality associated with these group characteristics as inequitable, and accordingly change the construct and focus of these group characteristics as analytical variables.

In addition to the need for clarifying the definition of health equity, part 2 makes further recommendations to *Healthy People 2010*. Most analyses of inequity in health states in the final review of *Healthy People 2000* (U.S. Department of Health and Human Services 1991) look only at death (National Center for Health Statistics 2001). While mortality provides the most robust information, part 2 has proven that health inequity analysis can be extended to health-adjusted quality of life. It is particularly disappointing that *Healthy People 2000* and *Healthy People 2010* rarely use the HALex given that the HALex was developed to monitor the health of Americans during the 1990s (Erickson, Wilson, and Shannon 1995) and *Healthy People 2010* claims the importance of looking at the health-adjusted quality of life.

For the wider use of the HALex in the assessment of the health of Americans, future work should acknowledge that the HALex is derived from self-reported activity limitation and self-perceived health questions. Should we assess population health based on a self-reported measure of health such as the HALex or on an 'objective' measure of health such as a medical diagnosis? Observation of the differences in the HALex between men and women in this study suggests the importance of this question. This study showed that in both 1990 and 1995, women's HALex was lower than men's in all age groups, except among 0–14 year olds both in 1990 and 1995, 45–64 year olds in 1990, and 65 year olds and older in 1995. In contrast, life expectancy was 7 years higher for women than men in 1990, and 6.4 years higher for women than men in 1995. In addition, the WHO reports that healthy life expectancy, which combines life expectancy and quality of life, was 4.1 years higher for women (71.3 years) than men (67.2 years) in 2002 (World Health Organization 2004). Is women's health status 'objectively' lower than men's, or do women perceive their health status as lower than men's? What if we discovered that women perceive the same, 'objective' health conditions lower than men. Should we then consider low perception to be a health problem? The issue of perception is not only limited to sex but also applies to socio-economic status, racial groups, or geographic location. The future work needs to investigate how much of the difference in the HALex is due to the difference in perception, and identify the appropriateness of using the HALex or any other self-reported measure of health in the assessment of population health.

Statistical and Clinical Significance of Health Inequity

As for most empirical studies, a statistical inference for the degree of health inequity estimated provided useful information in examining the change in health equity between 1990 and 1995. Difficulties still remain, however, in interpreting the results due to the 0–1 unit of the measurement of health (the HALex) and the measurement of health inequity (the Gini coefficient and the FGT measure). Understanding clinical significance is important especially when using such a large data set as the NHIS, by which statistical significance is often easily obtainable. Even with a good understanding of the construction of these measures, however, results expressed in the 0–1 unit do not allow intuitive interpretation but only two extreme values, zero and one. It is easy to understand how long one year of life is, but it is not obvious, for example, how bad the 0.02 HALex reduction or 0.001 increase in the Gini coefficient and the FGT measure might be. A further challenge is that we must understand these non-intuitive numbers from the population perspective. Although the 0.02 HALex reduction or 0.001 reduction in the Gini coefficient and the FGT measure might appear to be small from the individual perspective, they might indicate clinically significant change from the population perspective.

Cutler and Richardson estimated the health-adjusted quality of life for selected disease conditions using the 1989–91 NHIS (1997). They compared self-reported health for people with and without a particular condition, estimated the effect of each condition by an ordered probit model, normalized the estimated effect, and reported the normalized values as quality of life scores for particular conditions. According to their calculation, the quality of life score of a person who has no health problem but glaucoma is 0.97, and that of a person who only suffers from sinusitis is 0,93. Although the quality of life scores estimated by Cutler and Richardson and those based on the HALex are, strictly speaking, not comparable, the quality of life scores by Cutler and Richardson suggest a possible magnitude of clinical significance of my analyses. For example, using these figures, if we compare a population in which everybody is in full health and another population in which everybody has no health problems but glaucoma, health inequality measured by the health-adjusted quality of life is 0.03. Similarly, for the case of sinusitis, health inequality is 0.07. In my analysis using the Rawlsian difference principle, health equity worsened between 1990 and 1995 among the living young adult population (25–44 years old) by 0.03 in the HALex. Using a figure by Cutler and Richardson, roughly speaking, this result indicates that the degree of inequity we are talking about here is equivalent to the situation in which everybody was in full health in 1990 while everybody had nothing but glaucoma in 1995.

The use of the Gini coefficient and the FGT measure for health distribution is also premature. The Gini coefficient was developed and has been extensively used for income distributions. The Gini coefficient for income distribution in industrialized countries is around 0.3 (Luxembourg Income Study 2006). The Gini coefficients for the HALex for the living populations of all ages and both sexes in the United States in 1990 and 1995 were around 0.1. This means that, considering both income and health as a multi-purpose resource useful for any life plan, health is much more equally distributed than income.

Table 6.16 summarizes the Gini coefficient applied to health distribution including the ones used for the living population from part 2. Le Grand (1987) and Illsley and Le Grand (1987) used the Gini coefficient for life years, and their studies show that in the early 1980s, the Gini coefficients for life years ranged between 0.109 and 0.141 in selected developed countries. These figures are still lower than the Gini coefficients for income distribution. Although study years are not exactly comparable, the Gini coefficient for life years appears to be greater than the Gini coefficient for the HALex. Table 6.16 also indicates that the 0.005 difference in the Gini coefficient of the HALex between 1990 and 1995 among Americans of all ages and both sexes is roughly equiv-

Table 6.16
Application of the Gini coefficient to health distributions

Population	Year	Gini coefficient	Health variable	Source
England & Wales, male	1921	0.237	age-standardized	Illsley and
	1931	0.212	age-at-death	Le Grand (1987)
	1941	0.216		
	1951	0.147		
	1961	0.137		
	1971	0.132		
	1981	0.127		
	1983	0.125		
England & Wales, female	1921	0.185	age-standardized	Illsley and
	1931	0.167	age-at-death	Le Grand (1987)
	1941	0.170		
	1951	0.122		
	1961	0.116		
	1971	0.115		
	1981	0.110		
	1983	0.109		
Australia	1981	0.125	age-at-death	Le Grand (1987)
Canada	1982	0.125		
Denmark	1982	0.121		
Finland	1981	0.118		
France	1981	0.133		
Japan	1982	0.118		
Norway	1982	0.120		
Romania	1982	0.141		
United States	1982	0.138		
Japan, all ages, both sexes	1989	0.091	the HALex	Asada and
	1998	0.091		Ohkusa (2004)
Japan, all ages, male	1989	0.085		
	1998	0.086		
Japan, all ages, female	1989	0.095		
	1998	0.096		
U.S., all ages, both sexes	1990	0.092	the HALex	Part 2 of this
	1995	0.097		book
U.S., all ages, male	1990	0.087		
	1995	0.092		
U.S., all ages, female	1990	0.097		
	1995	0.101		

alent to the difference in the Gini coefficient of life years between the
United States and France in the early 1980s or the difference in the Gini
coefficient of age-standardized life years between 1971 and 1981 among
people in England and Wales of all ages and both sexes.

Interpretation of the FGT measure ($\alpha = 2$) is even more challenging
with no comparable figures available. Despite the multidimensional
concept of poverty, income is most often used as the indicator of
poverty. The FGT measure ($\alpha = 2$), therefore, has rarely been applied
for a health distribution.[15] In addition, there is a difference in setting
the threshold in poverty analysis and health inequity analysis: the minimally adequate level of health in analysis in part 2 is not set as at a lower
end of a distribution, as is often the case for poverty analysis. Unlike
the case of the Gini coefficient, the FGT measure ($\alpha = 2$) applied for
income distribution would not provide a meaningful figure as a reference for the analysis in part 2.

Despite a number of shortcomings and prematurity, I believe that the
analyses in this chapter show the importance of logical consistency from
conceptualizing health inequity to conducting its empirical analysis.
Many of the analyses in this chapter had the same conclusion – unfortunately, bad news – that health equity worsened between 1990 and
1995 in the United States. Even if analysis using different perspectives
on health equity reached different conclusions, however, that would not
have been a problem. Results of empirical analysis are always informative as long as analysts are sure that they measured what they had
intended to measure.

7 Conclusion

7.1 Summary

If we are worried about health distribution for moral reasons, and interested in measuring it, how should we go about it? This book aims to help academics and policy-makers who have such a concern. To meet this goal, this book proposes a framework for measuring health inequality reflecting moral concerns (part 1). The framework consists of the following three steps: (1) defining when a health distribution becomes inequitable – that is, of moral concern, (2) deciding on measurement strategies to operationalize a chosen concept of health equity, and (3) summarizing a health distribution into one number. This book also shows how the framework can be used in quantitative studies and policy-making (part 2). Did health equity improve in the United States between 1990 and 1995? Using the 1990 and 1995 National Health Interview Survey (NHIS), the foregoing chapter examined this question from different perspectives on health equity with measurement strategies developed in the framework. To conclude this book, I provide a brief summary of each chapter, and then indicate future health equity work before us.

Chapters 1 and 2 correspond to the first of the three steps of measuring health inequity: when does a health distribution become inequitable? Chapter 1 started by discussing the various reasons why we might be interested in health distribution, including describing how health is distributed, understanding its mechanisms, and being concerned about its moral implications. I argued that our ethical interest in health distribution distinguishes health inequality as a topic, and I operationally defined the moral dimension of health distribution as health inequity. I then examined different ethical reasons why we might be interested in health distribution. A variety of views are possible, and I summarized them into three categories: health is special, health equity plays an important role in the general pursuit of justice, and health inequality is an indicator of general social justice.

In chapter 2, these three ethical interests in health distribution were further developed into specific perspectives on health equity. I critically reviewed a variety of perspectives on health equity, often only intuitively discussed in the health sciences literature, in connection with philosophical discussions of equality and justice. I started by showing why the idea of strict equality in health outcome does not provide an attractive account of health equity. For this idea to become attractive, I continued, the strictness of this idea must be relaxed either by cause or level. As examples of perspectives on health equity focusing on certain causes, I critically reviewed the view of health inequity as health inequality caused by socio-economic status, whose reasoning can be connected to John Rawls's theory of justice as fairness (1971) and Michael Walzer's idea of spheres of justice (1983), the view of health inequity as health inequality caused by factors beyond individual control (Le Grand 1991; Whitehead 1992), and the view of health inequity as health inequality caused by factors amenable to human interventions used for health inequality measurement in *The World Health Report 2000* (Gakidou, Murray, and Frenk 2000; World Health Organization 2000a).

As examples of focusing on a certain level of health, I examined the view of health equity as satisfying the minimally adequate level of health, whose justification can be derived from Norman Daniels's normal species functioning idea (1985) and Martha Nussbaum's version of the capability approach (2000). In addition, I introduced the proposal by Amartya Sen (1998), and Daniels, Kennedy, and Kawachi (2000; 2004), in which we are not concerned about which health – by cause or level – we should focus on as the equalization target, but perceive a health distribution as a whole as an indicator of social justice.

Chapter 3 corresponds to the second of the three steps of measuring health inequity: what measurement choices can be made in measuring health inequity? I listed health measurement, the unit of time, and the unit of analysis as important measurement questions, whose answer should reflect both our ideas of health equity and such usual empirical considerations as data availability and technical feasibility. I argued that one of the fundamental values of health, health as a multi-purpose resource useful for any life plan, supports health as functionality, and functionality as capacity. I also showed that this focus of health in health equity analysis coincides with the focus of health in cutting-edge health status measures and, therefore, emphasized the importance of incorporating the development of health status measurement into the development of health equity measurement. I also argued for the importance of recognizing the health production process in defining health in health equity analysis: do we focus on health determinants, expectation, or outcome in health inequity analysis? I pointed out a number of difficulties in applying health expectation to health inequity analysis and advocated the use of health outcome in health inequity analysis. Finally, I discussed the implications of distinguishing a health state with or without medical technologies, non-human aids, human assistance, and accommodating environmental factors.

Adapting Dennis McKerlie's philosophical argument on equality and time (1989) to health equity analysis, I next examined the period of time within which we should seek health equity. I discussed three approaches to segment time for health inequity analysis: the whole-life approach, the life-stage approach, and the cross-sectional approach. Ideally, I argued, we should combine the whole-life approach and the life-stage approach for health equity analysis. A consensus has yet to be achieved, however, on how to value health at different stages of life and combine it as the whole-life experience. I therefore concluded that the life-stage approach is for now the most reasonable unit of time for health equity analysis.

Since the release of the controversial *World Health Report 2000* (World Health Organization 2000a), the unit of analysis has been the most widely discussed measurement choice in health inequity analysis. Is health inequity better measured across individuals, as Gakidou, Murray, and Frenk proposed (Murray, Gakidou, and Frenk 1999), or groups of individuals, as the vast majority of health science researchers have traditionally conducted? I argued against the view of Gakidou, Murray, and Frenk that the central characteristic dividing these two approaches is the presence of a normative position. Instead, I suggested three distinguishing characteristics: the question of among whom we want to seek health equity, comparability, and selective information by averaging. Furthermore, I argued that we can simultaneously examine health inequity across individuals and groups of individuals by using the subpopulation decomposition technique frequently employed by economists in the income inequality field.

Chapter 4 corresponds to the last of the three steps of measuring health inequity: how can a health distribution be summarized into one number? I argued at the beginning of the chapter that the summary process inevitably requires selection, suppression, and omission of certain information carried by a health distribution. I emphasized that the decision to select a specific aspect of health inequity information must be guided by principle, rather than, as often is the case, convenience. Building up the philosopher Larry Temkin's work (1993) and the axiomatic approach in income inequality literature and health inequality measurement literature, I identified five key questions that arise when summarizing a health distribution into one number: (A) comparison, (B) aggregation, (C) sensitivity to the mean, (D) sensitivity to the population size, and (E) subgroup considerations. I argued that the following properties are desirable for inequality measures used for health inequity analysis: (a) comparison between everyone's health and everyone's health (unless one has a particular interest in a specific person or group or a certain norm), (b) asymmetric weighting in terms of location (greater weights towards the lower tail of the distribution), but no weighting in terms of size of differences, (c) the intermediate inequality concept (which judges that the equal absolute addition reduces inequality while the equal proportional increase makes inequality bigger), (d) insensitivity to the population size, and (e) sensitivity to subgroup population size and decomposability by subgroup. I showed that among five popular health inequality measures used as examples in chapter 4 the Concentration Index and the Gini coefficient satisfy all of these characteristics, except (c), and suggested their good promise for health inequity analysis. I emphasized different ways in which subgroup decomposition is done in these measures – in the Gini coefficient overall health inequality is decomposed while in the Concentration Index group-related (for example, income-related) health inequality is decomposed.

Chapter 5 started by providing an overview of empirical illustration in part 2. A major objective of part 2, I argued, was to bridge health equity concepts developed in the previous chapters to empirical analyses. I stated the question that I was going to ask in part 2: did health equity improve in the United States between 1990 and 1995 from different perspectives on health equity developed in part 1? I also explained three methodological challenges that analyses in part 2 took up, namely, using a health status measure as the measurement of health, including the dead in the analyses, and making a statistical inference for the degree of health inequity estimated.

In addition, chapter 5 composed building blocks necessary for health inequity analyses in part 2. I described the 1990 and 1995 National Health Interview Survey. In addition, I explained measurement of health, measurement of health inequity, and the unit of time that I was going to use for the analyses. I emphasized that every measurement decision I made in the analyses in this chapter related to questions discussed in the previous chapters. Following discussion in chapter 3, for example, I selected a health status measure, the Health and Activity Limitation Index (HALex), as the measurement of health. Based on discussion in chapter 4, I decided to employ the Gini coefficient and a poverty measure, the Foster-Greer-Thorbecke (FGT) measure, as health inequity measures. In addition, reflecting examination of the unit of time and the unit of analysis in health inequity analysis in chapter 3, whenever deemed effective, I chose to employ the life-stage approach, and I analysed health inequity across individuals as well as groups of individuals by using the subpopulation decomposition technique.

Before conducting health inequity analyses, I presented a preliminary analysis of the average HALex in the United States between 1990 and 1995. My analysis showed that health status measures captured a different aspect of health than measures of life years: between 1990 and 1995, life expectancy increased in the United States, but the HALex on average stayed about the same. Moreover, women's HALex was lower than men's in both 1990 and 1995. I ended chapter 5 by asking how the assessment of health of Americans might change if one looked at the distribution of health rather than the average health.

This was exactly the question I asked in chapter 6. Did health equity improve in the United States between 1990 and 1995? I examined this question from four different perspectives on health equity developed in chapter 2. I first employed the view of health inequality as an indicator of social justice, in which a health distribution is considered to carry important information on how in general a society functions, and, therefore, all observing health inequalities are the analytic interest. With the second series of analyses, using the view of health inequity as health inequality associated with such a specific group characteristic as race, sex and gender, income, or education, I warned against the widespread tendency in the health sciences field to find that all health inequalities associated with any group characteristic are inequitable. The third equity perspective employed, the view of health inequity as health inequality caused by socio-economic status, is the most popular equity perspective in the health sciences field. Reflecting the discussion in chapter 2 on how this popular but intuitive equity perspective can be bridged to reach sound philosophical theories of equality and justice, I incorporated the Rawlsian difference principle (1971) and Walzer's view of dominance as unjust (1983) in the analysis. Finally, I adopted the view of health equity as satisfying the minimally adequate level of health inspired by Nussbaum's version of the capability approach (2000).

Chapter 6 subsequently discussed findings of the analyses. Despite a number of different perspectives on health equity used, analyses in chapter 6 showed that health equity in the United States had in most cases deteriorated between 1990 and 1995. Furthermore, employing the life-stage approach in the view of health inequality as an indicator of social justice, the Rawlsian difference principle, and the view of health equity as satisfying the minimally adequate level of health suggested that the deterioration was primarily due to that of young adults (25–44 years old). The only hopeful observation during this period was the improvement of health equity associated with race.

7.2 Future Work

Some questions raised in this book have been suspended. Others lead to further questions. They are left prematurely or completely open, not because they lack importance but because they suggest how profound a topic health inequity is. To conclude this book, I list some questions for future work on health inequity:

- *How Can We Pursue Health Equity in the Full Recognition of Cost Constraints?*
  This book introduced various perspectives on health equity. While most of them appear to be attractive if the sole focus is on equity in health, promoting health equity in the real world must be realized under cost constraints. How do we balance equity with resources? What perspective of health equity can provide reasonable guidance for improving health equity without bankrupting a society? Weighing the importance of these questions, economists argue that we should examine health equity always as equity-efficiency trade-offs within the social welfare framework. Throughout the book, I have maintained that it is premature to take this approach before clarifying the complex notion of health inequity. Once we have a clear understanding of health equity, to be of value in the real world, we must incorporate cost constraints.

• *Within What Population Is It Meaningful to Analyse Health Inequity?*
This book has defined a population as a collection of individuals or
groups. But is there a better definition of a population within which
analysis of health inequity is meaningful? This question relates to
the question of responsibility: who should be responsible for health
inequity observed? Using a country as a population is straightforward in this regard, as it appears to be legitimate to expect the
government of the country to be responsible for health inequity
observed within that country. Yet in this global age, is there any
good reason why the definition of a population should be limited to
a nation state? Conversely, in such federal states as the United States
and Canada, given that a regional government has more power than
the federal government in some area of people's lives, is it not more
meaningful to analyse health inequity within a state or province or
region rather than within a country?

• *Why Should We Focus on Health Outcomes Rather than Health Determinants in the Pursuit of Health Equity?*
In chapter 3, I introduced three focal points of health: health determinants, expectation, and outcomes. I argued that focusing on
health expectation causes various problems, but in the pursuit of
health equity is there any reason to favour health determinants over
outcomes or vice versa? One important question of this kind yet to
be answered is whether we judge a health distribution still inequitable when such health determinants as health care, socio-economic
factors, and environmental factors are equitably distributed.[1] Or,
can a health distribution still be inequitable when an equitable
system of health services is provided to all members of a society
(Musgrove 1986)? The answer to these questions will primarily
depend on whether we judge unequal health outcomes caused by
factors beyond human control to be inequitable.

• *How Best Do the Development of Health Status Measures and the Development of Health Inequity Measures Proceed Together?*
Without measuring health, one can never measure health inequity.
This book has shown a close relationship between the development
of health status measures and that of health inequity measures. The
discussion of health measurement in chapter 3 should give an
insight to the development of health status measures. For example,
the suggestion of distinguishing 'bare' health, medical technologies,

non-human aids, human assistance, and accommodating environmental factors would be particularly interesting. In addition to the
discussion in chapter 3, the use of the HALex in the empirical case
studies in part 2 indicated the need of reassessing self-reported
health status measures.

- *What is the Relationship between Health Inequity and the Population's
  Mean Health?*
  The goal of improving population health is now frequently considered to be twofold: increasing the mean population health and
  reducing health inequity. In this book, I have treated the mean and
  inequity as separate issues. Yet there are indications that we cannot
  treat considerations to the mean and inequity as completely separate. Examination of the construction of health inequity measures
  in chapter 4, for example, has made it clear that these are not
  entirely conceptually separate. In addition, if we were to use a
  cutting-edge health status measure in health inequity analysis,
  because of its construction, the health status measure would itself
  embed the mean value of health states in the population. What
  exactly is the relationship between health inequity and the population's mean health?

- *How Can We Best Deal with Relationships between Health and Other Goods?*
  Throughout this book, I have primarily isolated health from other
  important goods whose distributions are also of moral concern. In
  chapter 1, I discussed how the isolation of health could be justified
  if there was a good reason to believe health is special or more
  important than other valuable goods. The chapters that followed
  have shown that this is one of the fundamental questions in conceptualizing and measuring health inequity, and it haunts us at various
  steps in doing so. Future work is necessary to investigate relationships between health and other important goods and examine how
  special health is among them. To rephrase it as a policy question,
  how much should be spent in health as opposed to such other pro-
  grams as education, social security, and transportation?

- *What Is the Most Attractive Definition of Health Equity?*
  This book is intended to guide health inequity analysis showing
  various possible paths without claiming the best way to measure
  health inequity. Yet, investigating more critically such questions as

the above, what then is the most attractive definition of health equity?

- *Is There Any Way to Summarize Diverse Perspectives on Health Equity?*
  There may indeed be no single best perspective on health equity, or we may not be comfortable with the uniform perspective on health equity. Can we then find a way to summarize diverse views of health equity? Such an examination must go both to the conceptual and methodological levels. Conceptually, we must investigate distinct characteristics each equity perspective holds and relationships between different perspectives. Methodologically, we must examine whether different aspects of health inequity can be summarized by a 'super' health inequity measure. For example, in chapter 6 I conducted empirical analysis one by one adopting a different perspective on health equity at a time. Can we summarize different perspectives together? Can we say that health equity is better when more aspects of health equity improve, for example, health equity associated with race, sex or gender, income, and education?

One fascinating fact about the topic of health equity is that it is excitingly multidisciplinary, as vividly shown in a wide range of previous work from which this book was drawn. Researchers from different disciplines must constructively learn from each other and creatively synthesize their ideas. Only in a dynamic, collaborative effort can we further advance our understanding in health equity.

Appendix A:
Five Popular Health Inequality Measures

A.1. The Range Measures

The range group includes such measures as differences, ratio, and the Shortfalls in Achievement.[1] See the examples of the two-group population in figure A.1.

The difference in the group average health-adjusted life years (HALYs) between Group A and B can be expressed differently by these range measures. The absolute difference measure suggests that there are 30 HALYs difference between A and B, and the ratio measure that B's HALYs are twice as long as A's. In the Shortfalls in Achievement, suppose we set a norm at 50 HALYs, then the Shortfalls in Achievement tells that A's HALYs are 20 HALYs lower than the set norm, 50 HALYs. By setting a norm, the Shortfalls in Achievement is concerned about how far behind a group is from the norm, and it pays no attention to the distribution above the norm. It is possible to express the Shortfalls in Achievement in relative terms using the lowest figure possible in a given comparison (United Nations Development Program 2001, 240). For example, if we set the lowest possible HALYs as 20 HALYs, the Shortfalls in Achievement for A works out thus:

$$\frac{\text{actual value} - \text{lowest value}}{\text{norm} - \text{lowest value}} = \frac{30 - 20}{50 - 20} = 0.33.$$

Although the range measures can also be used for individuals, in the health inequality context, they are primarily used for comparison between groups, as this example illustrates. The health of each group is often expressed in rates (e.g., mortality or morbidity rates), and corresponding range measures are called the rate differences and the rate ratios.

Figure A.1   Range measures

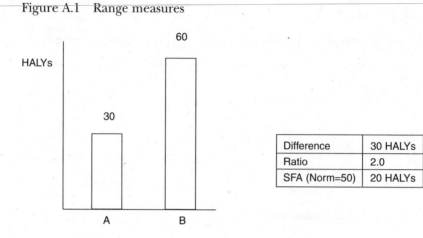

Difference	30 HALYs
Ratio	2.0
SFA (Norm=50)	20 HALYs

A.2. The Concentration Index and the Generalized Concentration Index

The Concentration Index is best understood with the Concentration Curve. Imagine that we horizontally line up socio-economic groups from the lowest to the highest and vertically plot these groups' health share, for example, the cumulative percentage of HALYs (Figure A.2).

The resulting curve AC is called a Concentration Curve for health, and the Concentration Index is twice the area between the diagonal line and the Concentration Curve (the shaded area in figure A.2). The Concentration Index moves between minus one and plus one, with zero as the most equal situation. The Concentration Index takes a positive value when the Concentration Curve is below the diagonal line, and a negative value above it. The Concentration Index minus one means that all the population's health is concentrated in people who belong to the socially most disadvantaged group, and plus one, it is concentrated in those who belong to the socially most advantaged group. The Concentration Index multiplied by the population's mean health level is called the Generalized Concentration Index, and unlike its original, it is insensitive to the equal addition (Clarke et al. 2002; Wagstaff, Paci, and van Doorslaer 1991).

Although these measures were developed for group data, it is possible to use them for individual data. Note, however, that even in this case individuals are placed in terms of social rank by these measures.

Figure A.2   The Concentration Curve

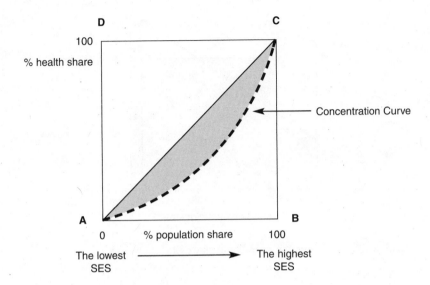

The Concentration Indices for individuals (Ci) and groups (Cg) are arithmetically expressed as follows (Kakwani, Wagstaff, and van Doorslaer 1997):

$$Ci = \frac{2}{n\mu} \sum_{i=1}^{n} y_i R_i - 1,$$

where y_i represents the ill-health score of the ith individual, and R_i is the relative social rank of the ith person (from the most disadvantaged to the advantaged).

$$Cg = \frac{2}{\mu} \sum_{t=1}^{T} f_t \mu_t R_t - 1,$$

where μ_t $(t=1,...,T)$ is the ill-health rate of the tth socio-economic group and f_t is the population share of the tth socio-economic group.

A.3. The Slope Index of Inequality and the Relative Index of Inequality

Although I do not discuss these two measures in the text, it is worth explaining these measures for their similarities to the Concentration

Figure A.3   The Slope Index of Inequality

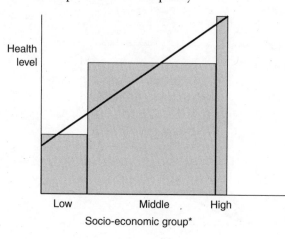

Socio-economic group*

*The width represents the population share of each group.

Index and the generalized Concentration Index. The Slope Index of Inequality is the coefficient of the weighted least squares regression based on the proportional size of each subgroup in figure A.3 (Pamuk 1985, 1988). The Slope Index of Inequality takes absolute values, for example, people on average expect to earn five more HALYs if they move up one socio-economic group. When the Slope Index of Inequality is divided by the population's mean level of health, it is called the Relative Index of Inequality, insensitive to the equal proportional change.

Wagstaff and his colleagues showed similarities between the Slope Index of Inequality and the Generalized Concentration Index, and the Relative Inequality Index and the Concentration Index (1991). The relationship between the Relative Inequality Index (RII) and the Concentration Index (CI), for example, is shown as

$$RII\left(\frac{\beta}{\mu}\right) = \frac{CI}{2\mathrm{var}(R)} \, ,$$

where R is a relative social rank variable. Given the similarities, according to them, there is no significant reason to choose between the Relative Inequality Index and the Concentration Index, or the Slope Index of Inequality and the generalized Concentration Index. They recommend the use of the Relative Inequality Index (or the Concentration

Figure A.4   The Lorenz Curve

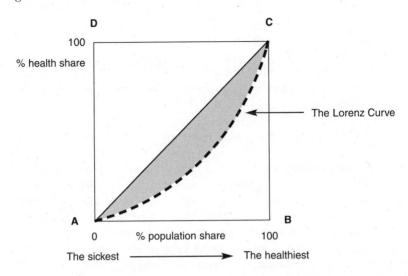

Index) as they believe insensitivity to equal proportional change is a desirable property for health inequality measures (see the section on sensitivity to the mean in chapter 4).

A.4. The Gini Coefficient

It is easiest to understand the Gini coefficient by defining the Lorenz Curve first. If used for health distribution, the Lorenz curve can be illustrated as figure A.4.

The Gini coefficient and the Concentration Index originate from the same Lorenz Curve concept, and the similarity is obvious. Unlike the Concentration Index, however, the order in which individuals line up horizontally is according to a health ranking from the sickest to the healthiest. The resulting curve AC is called the Lorenz Curve. When the population is perfectly equal, the Lorenz Curve is diagonal, AC. When the population is most unequal, that is, one person is alive with or without some health-related quality and all others are dead, the Lorenz Curve follows AB and BC. The Gini coefficient is the shaded area in the graph divided by the triangle, ABC. It can take a value between zero when the Lorenz Curve is diagonal, thus, perfectly equal, and one when the Lorenz Curve goes AB and BC, the most unequal.

Arithmetically, the Gini coefficient (G) is shown to be the same as the relative mean difference, and expressed as

$$G = \frac{1}{2} \sum_{i=1}^{n} \sum_{j=1}^{n} \frac{|y_i - y_j|}{n^2 \mu},$$

where the population of interest holds n people, y_i is the health of individual i, y_j is the health of individual j, and the average level of health in the population is μ.

A.5. The WHO Health Inequality Index

In *The World Health Report 2000*, Gakidou, Murray, and Frenk launched the WHO's health inequality project by measuring equality in survival of children less than two years of age (Gakidou, Murray, and Frenk 2000; World Health Organization 2000a). Thus, to be precise, its health inequality measure is only for child survival, but here we assume that the same measurement will also be used beyond childhood, as Gakidou, Murray, and Frenk themselves intend to do in the future. The WHO health inequality index is as follows:

$$\text{Equality of Child Survival} = \left[1 - \frac{\sum_{i=1}^{n} \sum_{j=1}^{n} |y_i - y_j|^3}{2n^2 \mu^{0.5}} \right],$$

where y is the survival time of a given child, μ is the mean survival time across children, and n is the number of children in the population.

Pay attention to the shaded part of the equation. The similarity with the Gini coefficient is obvious. In section 4.4 in chapter 4 I discussed differences between these two measures. In the WHO health inequality index, perfect equality is represented by one. With the exponential form, unlike the Gini coefficient, the degree of inequality can be more than one. Gakidou, Murray, and Frenk say that no country in their analysis ever yielded inequalities more than one, thus their equality measure never reached below zero, suggesting that 'zero can be interpreted as a degree of inequality that is worse than has been seen in any country measured directly or estimated indirectly to date' (World Health Organization 2000a, 147).

Appendix B:
Intermediate Inequality in the WHO
Health Inequality Index

The WHO health inequality index adopts the intermediate inequality concept based on the survey respondents' perceptions about the sensitivity to the mean level (Gakidou, Murray, and Frenk 2001). The WHO questionnaire presented two populations (like Population A and D in the bottom two illustrations of figure 4.5a, in chapter 4, note 22) and asked which of the two populations has greater health inequality. It used three patterns with positive and negative health measures (life expectancy, probability of survival, and probability of death). Based on the respondents' answers, Gakidou, Murray, and Frenk judged that 54% of the total respondents thought that inequality measures should reflect relative difference while 46% of the respondents absolute difference. Based on these results, they decided to adopt the intermediate inequality concept in its measurement.

One can incorporate the intermediate inequality concept in the measurement in various ways. The procedure that Gakidou, Murray, and Frenk took was to decide the value of the exponent of the mean. The WHO health inequality index (W) is as follows:[2]

$$W = \frac{\sum_{i=1}^{n} \sum_{j=1}^{n} |y_i - y_j|^{\alpha}}{2n^2 \mu^{\beta}},$$

where y is the health of an individual, n is the population size, and μ is the population's mean health level. As we saw in the section dealing with the weighting issues, Gakidou, Murray, and Frenk decided to take $\alpha = 3$. They opted for $\beta = 0.54$ reflecting that 54% of people thought that inequality measures should reflect relative difference.

Table B1
Hypothetical populations

	Population F	Population G	Population H	Population I
	Perfect equality		Equal proportional increase (H = 2 x G)	Equal absolute addition (I = G + 10)
Person 1	50	20	40	30
Person 2	50	30	60	40
Person 3	50	40	80	50
Person 4	50	40	80	50
Person 5	50	50	100	60
Mean	50	36	72	46

To simplify the argument, let us first look at the case of $\alpha = 1$, that is, no weight is attached to each health difference compared within the population. β can take a value between zero and one. When β is zero, the inequality measure is insensitive to the equal absolute difference (translation invariant); when β is one, the measure is insensitive to the equal proportional difference (scale invariant). Any values in between reflect the intermediate inequality concept: the equal absolute addition reduces inequality, while the equal proportional increase makes inequality bigger. An in-between value β represents how much health inequality reduction or increase occurs, or, in Kolm's terminology, how much 'left' or 'right' our judgment is. An example might help understand the point. I created four hypothetical populations, each of which contains five people (table B.1). We are here interested in inequality in life years across five people in each population. Life years of everyone in Population F is fifty years, so Population F is perfectly equal in terms of life years. Population G presents some inequality in life years. Life years of everyone in Population H are twice longer than life years of everyone in Population G. In other words, the differences between Population H and G are equiproportional. Everyone in Population I has ten years longer life years than Population G, thus, the differences between Population F and I are equal absolute difference. I first calculated the formula W with $\alpha = 1$ and different values for β from zero to one. Table B.2 summarizes the results. W equals to zero when applied to a population with perfect equality (Popu-

Table B2
Translation invariance, intermediate inequality, and scale invariance ($\alpha = 1$)

β	Population F	Population G	Population H	Population I
	Perfect equality		Equal proportional increase (H = 2 x G)	Equal absolute addition (I = G + 10)
0	0	5.60	11.20	5.60
0.2	0	2.73	4.76	2.60
0.4	0	1.34	2.02	1.21
0.5	0	0.93	1.32	0.83
0.54	0	0.81	1.11	0.71
0.6	0	0.65	0.86	0.56
0.8	0	0.32	0.37	0.26
1	0	0.16	0.16	0.12

$\beta = 0.54$ is the value chosen by Gakidou, Murray, and Frenk (2001).
When $\beta = 0$, W is translation invariant; when $0 < \beta < 1$, W suggests intermediate inequality; when $\beta = 1$, W is scale invariant.

lation F), and the larger the W is, the greater inequality is. Comparing Population G and H, when $\beta = 1$, equal proportional increase has no effect on the degree of inequality, while β values between zero and 0.8 express different degrees of how much the equal proportional increase makes inequality bigger. Comparing Population G and I, when $\beta = 0$, equal absolute addition does not change the degree of inequality, but β values between 0.2 and 1.0 suggest different degrees of how much the equal absolute addition reduces inequality. In summary, when $\beta = 0$, W is translation invariant; when β takes values between 0.2 and 0.8, W has the property of intermediate inequality; and $\beta = 1$, W is scale invariant. Further research is necessary to decide which specific value β should take and in what way we can investigate this question.

Next, I calculated different values for β between zero and one using the WHO health inequality index's value, $\alpha = 3$, that is, each difference of health is cubed and added (table B.3). Note that, despite the claim by Gakidou, Murray, and Frenk (2001, 5), when $\beta = 1$, W is not scale invariant, and instead suggests intermediate inequality. Why? Simple mathematics can show this point clearly. Let us look at the calculation

Table B3

Translation invariance, intermediate inequality, and scale invariance ($\alpha = 3$)

	Population F	Population G	Population H	Population I
β	Perfect equality		Equal proportional increase (H = 2 x G)	Equal absolute addition (I = G + 10)
0	0	2240	17920	2240
0.2	0	1094	7619	1042
0.4	0	534	3239	484
0.5	0	373	2112	330
0.54	0	323	1780	283
0.6	0	261	1377	225
0.8	0	127	585	105
1	0	62	249	49

$\beta = 0.54$ is the value chosen by Gakidou, Murray, and Frenk (2001).
When $\beta = 0$, W is translation invariant; when $0 < \beta < 1$, W suggests intermediate inequality.

for the degree of inequality in Population G and H in table B.2. The health level of each of the five people in Population H is proportionally increased from each person's health in Population A. When $\alpha = 1$ and $\beta = 1$, the degree of inequality in Population G and H is the same. But when $\alpha = 3$ and $\beta = 1$, it is not. Let subscript G stand for values in Population G, and subscript H for values in Population H:

$$y_{Hi} = y_{Gi} \times 2,$$
$$y_{Hj} = y_{Gj} \times 2,$$

$$\left| y_{Hi} - y_{Hj} \right| = \left| y_{Gi} - y_{Gj} \right| \times 2.$$

Health inequality in Population H measured by the WHO's health inequality measure is as follows:

When $\alpha = 1$

$$W_H = \frac{\sum_{i=1}^{n} \sum_{j=1}^{n} \left| y_{Hi} - y_{Hj} \right|}{2 n_H^2 \mu_H^\beta} = \frac{\sum_{i=1}^{n} \sum_{j=1}^{n} \left(\left| y_{Gi} - y_{Gj} \right| \times 2 \right)}{2 n_G^2 \mu_G^\beta \times 2}$$

$$= \frac{\left(\sum_{i=1}^{n} \sum_{j=1}^{n} |y_{Gi} - y_{Gj}| \right) \times 2}{2 n_G^2 \mu_G^\beta \times 2} = W_G.$$

When $\alpha = 3$

$$W_H = \frac{\sum_{i=1}^{n} \sum_{j=1}^{n} |y_{Hi} - y_{Hj}|^3}{2 n_H^2 \mu_H^\beta} = \frac{\sum_{i=1}^{n} \sum_{j=1}^{n} (|y_{Gi} - y_{Gj}| \times 2)^3}{2 n_G^2 \mu_G^\beta \times 2}$$

$$= \frac{\left(\sum_{i=1}^{n} \sum_{j=1}^{n} |y_{Gi} - y_{Gj}| \right)^3 \times 2^3}{2 n_G^2 \mu_G^\beta \times 2} = W_G \times 2^2.$$

Simple enough, the equiproportional factor, 2, is not cancelled out when $\alpha = 3$. Gakidou, Murray, and Frenk intended to use its health inequality index, W, as an intermediate inequality measure with $\beta = 0.54$, and, as table B.2 shows, this itself is valid. Yet this example suggests a complex relationship between the five questions that arises upon summarizing a distribution into one number, in this case between the sensitivity to the mean and aggregation. Depending on the choice of weight, one cannot simply raise the mean to the power of some number between zero and one to express the sensitivity to the mean.

Another point to note in tables B.2 and B.3 is that the degree of inequality is hardly bounded by zero and one. When Gakidou, Murray, and Frenk first used its health inequality index for equality in child survival under two years of age, it gave an impression that its measure takes a value between zero and one, the latter expressing the perfect equality. As pointed out by Szwarcwald (2002), this is 'by chance' due to small numbers of child survival years it used. Depending on the value range of the chosen health measure, W can take any values greater than zero. This may not be a problem if the meaning is clear, but the zero-one boundary of a measure like the Gini coefficient gives an easy interpretation.

Appendix C:
The Dead Imputation

A cross-sectional survey only collects information on the living. I impute the number of the dead and include them in my analysis of distribution of health. The most straightforward imputation of the dead involves calculating the number of people who died between their births and the time of the survey. This strategy unfortunately suffers from technical and conceptual difficulties. Although it is theoretically possible to trace back a number of the dead from the vital statistics, the quality of the data may be questionable. Also, adjusting the vital statistics for migration of multiple years will be cumbersome, if not impossible. Moreover, even if we could obtain good quality vital statistics and adjust them perfectly for migration, the results of this sample of the living and the dead combined would not be of much use for policy-making. Some of the dead in this sample have 'just died,' that is, their deaths occurred last year, while others among the dead have been dead for many years. Adding deaths occurring over many years to the cross-sectional living population contributes a confusing mixture of birth cohort and cross-sectional perspectives.

Thus, I instead focus on deaths occurring around the survey years. Using the mortality rate of each age published in the complete life tables for the United States in 1990 and 1995, one can compute how many people in the living sample of 1990 and 1995 would be dead in the following years. A complete life table provides information for every single year of age, while an abridged life table only offers information with such age intervals as five or ten years. To estimate how many people in a living sample might be dying for the coming year following the survey year, a complete life table is necessary. Estimation of a complete life table requires more resource and time than an abridged life table,

Figure C.1   The dead imputation

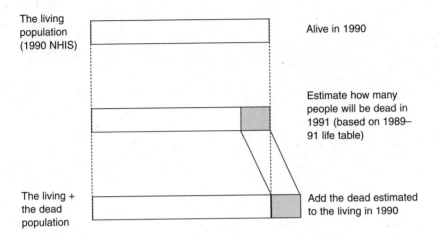

and until 1995, a complete life table for the U.S. population had only been constructed on a decennial basis. Since 1996, it has been constructed every year (Anderson, 1999).

Figure C.1 illustrates this dead imputation procedure with the example of the survey year of 1990. For the dead imputation of the 1990 NHIS living sample, I use the 1989–91 complete life tables for U.S. men and women (National Center for Health Statistics 1997) No complete annual U.S. life table is available for 1995, so I use the 1996 complete life tables (Anderson 1999) for the U.S. men and women as approximations for 1995.

A drawback of this method is that a number of imputed deaths will always be smaller than the actual number of deaths. This is because the mortality rates used in this method are not adjusted for health status, or as commonly known in demography, 'frailty.' The results in chapter 6, therefore, should be regarded as being biased towards the healthy.

The aforementioned dead imputation works for a cross-sectional survey with the simple random sampling. But further considerations are necessary when using surveys with other sampling methods. This is the case for the NHIS, which employs the complex survey design. For a point estimate, it is possible to impute a population frequency weight for each dead using the weighted and unweighted living populations of the NHIS: how many deaths in the target population are represented by a single dead person imputed. It is not possible, however, to obtain a standard error for a point estimate of any statistic using the dead. The aforementioned dead imputation only uses information of age and sex of the dead and does not provide any survey design information for them. I therefore only present point estimates, that is, degrees of health inequity, in the health inequity analyses including the dead.

Appendix D:
The Gini Coefficient

D.1. The Scale and Translation Invariant Gini Coefficient

How different are the degrees of inequality obtained by the scale invariant Gini coefficient and a modified Gini coefficient with the intermediate inequality concept? A quick way to examine this question is to compare degrees of inequality by the usual scale-invariant Gini coefficient (G) and the Gini coefficient modified so as to become translation invariant (G'):

$$G = \frac{1}{2} \sum_{i=1}^{n} \sum_{j=1}^{n} \frac{|y_i - y_j|}{n^2 \mu} \ ,$$

$$G' = \frac{1}{2} \sum_{i=1}^{n} \sum_{j=1}^{n} \frac{|y_i - y_j|}{n^2 \mu} \cdot \mu = \frac{1}{2} \sum_{i=1}^{n} \sum_{j=1}^{n} \frac{|y_i - y_j|}{n^2}.$$

Recall that the intermediate inequality concept lies between the translation and scale invariance. Thus, measuring health inequality by G and G', one would obtain the two extreme results. How different are the degrees of inequality obtained by these two measures? Comparing them, one can see how different the degree of health inequality might be if the Gini coefficient was modified and applied to the intermediate inequality concept.

Now I call readers' attention to the theoretical property and actual behaviour of an inequality measure. As I argued in chapter 4, when we look at any difference (or change) between the means in populations compared, it is important to know in what way the means are different. I introduced two stylized mean differences, the equal absolute difference and the equiproportional difference, and investigated the ques-

Table D.1
Scale and translation invariant Gini coefficient

Age group (years)	Mean HALex	Gini coefficient (scale invariant)	Gini coefficient x mean (translation invariant)	Difference
0–14	0.93	0.048	0.045	0.003
15–24	0.92	0.056	0.052	0.005
25–44	0.90	0.072	0.065	0.007
44–64	0.82	0.127	0.104	0.023
65+	0.73	0.183	0.134	0.049

tion of the sensitivity to the mean based on these two stylized views. The difference between the means we observe in real life, however, rarely fits to either of these stylized mean differences. As much as we understand the theoretical sensitivity to the mean of an inequality measure at hand, it is also important to know how that inequality measure behaves with actual data of interest.

Table D.1 and Figure D.1 present the mean HALex, the scale-variant Gini coefficient, and the translation variant Gini coefficient of five age groups (0–14, 15–24, 25–44, 45–64, 65+ years old) of the living population in the 1990 NHIS. All values are appropriately weighted. Both scale- and translation-invariant Gini coefficients give the same description that inequality increases as the mean HALex lowers in older ages. The difference is how much more inequality exists at the lower means. The scale-invariant Gini coefficient suggests more inequality at lower means than the translation-invariant Gini coefficient, and the lower the mean, the more discrepancy there is. Note that the Gini coefficient with the intermediate inequality concept, if successfully adapted, would take values between those of the scale and translation-invariant Gini coefficients. Differences of 0.003–0.049 between degrees of inequality calculated by the scale- and translation-invariant Gini coefficient might appear to be small. But until the Gini coefficient is more widely used in health inequity analysis, it is difficult to assess how much concern we should have for these differences. At the current limited state of application, it seems sensible to stay with the ordinary, scale-invariant Gini coefficient.

Figure D.1   Scale and translation invariant Gini coefficient

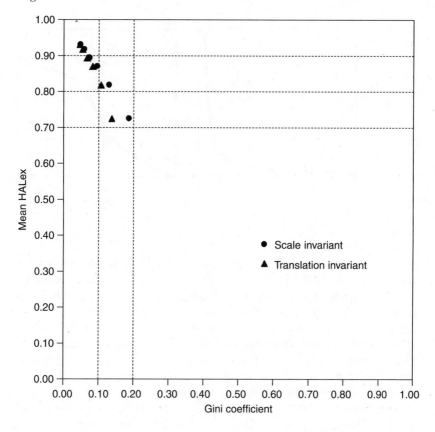

D.2. Application of the Gini Coefficient to the HALex

The Gini coefficient has extensively been used for income distribution. Income takes values between negative infinity and positive infinity.[3] The HALex, on the other hand, takes values between zero and one. Before applying the Gini coefficient to the HALex, whose boundary is considerably different from that of income, we need to investigate whether further consideration is necessary.

As with many health status measures, the HALex suffers from the ceiling effect, that is, a large majority of people in a population con-

Figure D.2   The ceiling and 'anchor' effects of the HALex

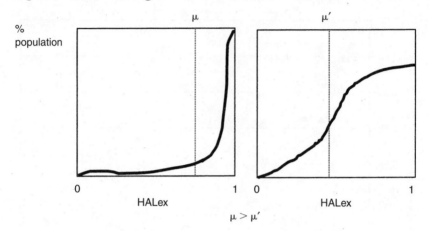

centrate on the value of one and values just below one. In chapter 3, I argued that the ceiling effect does not cause any concern in terms of assessing equity of health as a multi-purpose resource: a health status measure such as the HALex focuses on the right aspect of health reflecting our value of health as a multi-purpose resource, and the ceiling effect merely suggests that more people possess more rather than less of that resource. Applying the Gini coefficient, however, to numbers with the characteristic of the ceiling effect requires caution.

It is important to notice that the minimum value of the HALex is almost always 0.1 and the maximum value of the HALex is almost always 1.0 in a living population. Unless a population or subpopulation is defined by health status, there are always some in full health and others in a very poor health condition in a given population. This is a notable difference between health distribution and income distribution. Accordingly, unless a population or subpopulation is defined by health status, the HALex values are anchored at 0.1 and 1.0.[4] In addition, in most populations or subpopulations we examine, we almost always observe the ceiling effect of the HALex. When the ceiling effect and the "anchor" effect come together, the mean HALex and inequality of the HALex show a consistent relationship: the lower the mean, the greater the inequality (Figure D.2).

In general, the population's mean health and health distribution do not have a consistent relationship. And if they do, they are usually thought of as going in the opposite direction: improving the mean health and increasing health equity are often considered as a difficult trade-off in population health policy-making. Because of the combination of the ceiling and anchor effects, in examination of population health applying the Gini coefficient to the HALex, the two population health goals accidentally move together. To decide whether this phenomenon is a problem, we need further research.

One way to investigate the relationship between the mean and the Gini coefficient of the HALex distribution is to find out the functional form of the probability density function that can best fit the HALex distribution. Once we obtain the functional form, we will be able to examine mathematically the relationship between the mean and the Gini coefficient. In the income inequality field, economists have extensively studied what probability density function can best describe a distribution of income or wealth, and suggested a number of possibilities, including the log-normal distribution, the beta distribution, and the gamma distribution (Bandourian 2000). In the field of health inequality, Gakidou and King used the beta-binomial distribution to model the probability of child survival from birth to two years of age (2002). In addition to being able to see a distribution in a continuous manner (Deaton 1997, 169–71), understanding the functional form of the best-fit distribution is useful, for example, when one is interested in drawing a statistical inference for the degree of health inequality estimated using the asymptotic properties (Litchfield 1999), or when the distribution of interest is unobservable (the case for Gakidou and King). Discussion in this appendix suggests that investigation of the function that best fits the HALex distribution will also help us determine a relationship between the mean and the Gini coefficient inherent in the shape of the HALex distribution.

D.3. Statistical Inference for the Gini Coefficient by Bootstrapping

Bootstrap is a simulation method only using data at hand, and with a few assumptions, it can provide a statistical inference for any statistic. The theory is simple.[5] Suppose we observe a random sample $\{X_1, X_2, ..., X_n\}$ from an unknown probability distribution F and we are interested in estimating a parameter of F, $\theta(F)$. The empirical distribution function $\hat{F}$ is defined to be the distribution that puts probability $1/n$ on each data point observed. A bootstrap sample $\{X_1^*, X_2^*, ..., X_n^*\}$ is an independent random sample consisting of n data values drawn with replacement from the empirical distribution $\hat{F}$. We can obtain an estimate of the parameter $\hat{\theta}^*$ $(X_1^*, X_2^*, ..., X_n^*)$ from this bootstrap sample. We repeatedly select a bootstrap sample B times, and obtain B independent estimates of the parameter $\hat{\theta}_1^*(\hat{F}), \hat{\theta}_2^*(\hat{F}), ..., \hat{\theta}_B^*(\hat{F})$ These values can then be used to estimate, for example, bias, the standard error by the sample standard deviation of the B replications, and confidence intervals. In the following, I use the percentile method to calculate 95% confidence intervals by looking at 5th percentile and 95th percentile of $\hat{\theta}^*$'s distribution.[6]

It has been shown that when B approaches infinity, the accuracy with which the bootstrap distribution estimates increases. A large number of B, however, comes with the computational cost. A consensus is yet to be achieved as to how many B is enough for what purpose. There are ad hoc rules regarding the number B, and it is generally suggested that 50–200 replications are enough for robust estimates of standard errors (Efron and Tibshirani 1993) but more than 1000 replications may be necessary for estimating confidence intervals (Heinrich 1998). For the health inequity analyses in chapter 6, I estimate confidence intervals for the Gini coefficient estimated, thus, I use 2000 replications.

The aforementioned application of the bootstrap responds to the challenge of drawing a statistical inference for the Gini coefficient but does not account for the complex survey design. The bootstrap method as described above assumes independence of observations, thus, without modification, it cannot be legitimately applied to data using the complex survey design. Modification of the original bootstrap has been suggested for variance estimation of the complex survey design.[7] For the analyses of health equity using the Gini coefficient in chapter 6, I used the two-stage With-Replacement Bootstrap (BWR), in which a bootstrap sample is randomly selected with replacement in two stages.[8] See figure D.3 for histograms of the Gini coefficient distributions based on 2000 replications using the two-stage BWR method.

D.4. Subgroup Decomposition of the Gini Coefficient

Suppose we have subpopulation $k = 1, 2, ..., n$. Decomposition of the Gini coefficient (G) by subpopulation can be expressed as follows:[9]

$$G = G_B + \sum a_k G_k + G_O ,$$

Figure D.3   Histograms of the Gini coefficient distributions, based on 2000 replications (Living population, United States)

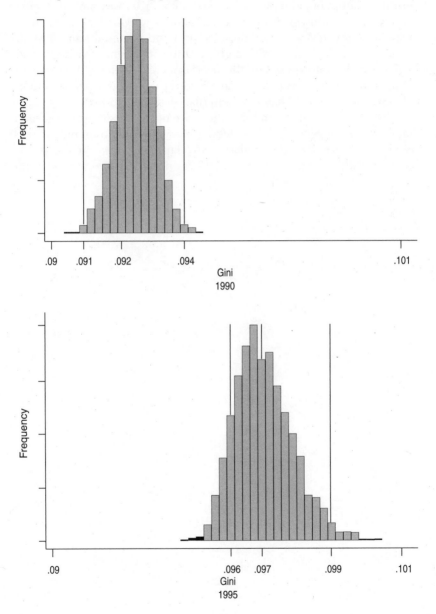

where G_B is the between-group Gini coefficient, calculated under the assumption that everybody's health in subpopulation k is the average health of subpopulation k. G_k is the Gini coefficient within subpopulation k. Each within-group Gini coefficient is weighted by population share and health share of subpopulation k, and its sum for all subpopulations $\sum a_k G_k$ is the total within-group Gini coefficient. G_O is a residual, which can be interpreted as the overlap Gini coefficient. When subpopulations do not overlap, G_O equals to zero. Note that when subpopulations are identical, that is, subpopulations perfectly overlap, G_O also equals to zero.[10] Unless subpopulations are perfectly identical, a greater value of G_O suggests a higher degree of overlap of subpopulations.[11] A higher degree of subpopulation overlap indicates that the group characteristic does not have much effect on the way the good – in our case, health – is distributed.

Appendix E:
The Foster-Greer-Thorbecke (FGT) Measure

E.1. The FGT Measure ($\alpha = 0, 1, 2$)

The FGT measure is defined as follows:

$$P_\alpha = \frac{1}{N} \sum_{i=1}^{n} \left(\frac{z - y_i}{z} \right)^\alpha ,$$

where $y = (y_1, y_1, ..., y_N)$ is a vector of health in increasing order, z is the threshold line, $z - y_i$ is the health shortfalls of the ith individual, N is the total population, and n is the total number of those who below the threshold. α is a measure of the sensitivity to the health gap. The larger the α is, the more weight is assigned to sicker people below the threshold.

When $\alpha = 0$,

$$P_0 = \frac{n}{N} ,$$

P_0 is the head-count ratio and measures the proportion of people below the threshold in the population. P_0 takes values between 0 and 1, suggesting, respectively, no one is below the threshold and everyone is below the threshold.

When $\alpha = 1$,

$$P_1 = \frac{1}{N} \sum_{i=1}^{n} \frac{z - y_i}{z} ,$$

P_1 is the health-gap index and measures the average shortfall of people below the threshold over the whole population, expressed as a ratio to the threshold. It asks what proportion of the minimally adequate level

of health people below that level lack on average over the whole population. $P_1 = 0.15$, for example, means that the average health gap, when
spreading both above and below the threshold, is equivalent to 15% of
the value of the minimally adequate level of health. P_1 takes values
between 0 and 1, suggesting, respectively, no shortfall at all (i.e., no one
is below the minimally adequate level) and 100% shortfall (i.e., everyone in the population is dead, and therefore, everyone is below the minimally adequate level of health). P_1 does not take account of how many
people are below the line, but on average how far off those who below
the line are.

When $\alpha = 2$,

$$P_2 = \frac{1}{N} \sum_{i=1}^{n} \left(\frac{z - y_i}{z} \right)^2 \qquad \text{(2a)}$$

$$= H[G^2 + (1-G)^2 C_p^2] \qquad \text{(2b)}.$$

Where

$$H = \frac{n}{N},$$

$$G = \sum_{i=1}^{n} \frac{z - y_i}{nz},$$

$$C_p^2 = \sum_{i=1}^{n} \frac{(\bar{y}_p - y_i)^2}{n y_p^{-2}} \quad \text{where } \bar{y}_p = \sum_{i=1}^{n} \frac{y_i}{n}.$$

P_2 is the squared health-gap index, a weighted sum of health gaps with
the weight of a proportionate health gap itself (2a). P_2 is the combination of the head-count ratio, the health gap index, and the squared
Coefficient of Variation among those below the threshold (2b), therefore, sensitive to the inequality among those who below the threshold.
P_2 takes values between 0 and 1, suggesting, respectively, no one is below
the threshold, and everyone is dead and therefore below the threshold.
Smaller values between 0 and 1 suggest a greater achievement of the
minimally adequate level of health but do not provide intuitive interpretation like P_0 and P_1.

E.2. The Foster-Greer-Thorbecke (FGT) measure vs the Sen-Shorrocks-Thon (SST) Measure

Which of the measurements, the FGT measure or the SST measure, should we use for the analysis adopting the view of health equity as satisfying the minimally adequate level of health? The discussion below is somewhat lengthy but shows how this question can be answered by principle rather than convenience.

The SST measure is defined as follows:[12]

$$P_{SST} = P_0 \, P_1{}^p \, (1 + \hat{G}^p),$$

where $P_0 = \dfrac{n}{N}$ is the head-count ratio, $P_1{}^p = \dfrac{1}{N} \displaystyle\sum_{i=1}^{N} \dfrac{z - y_i}{z}$ is the health gap index, and $\hat{G}^p$ is the Gini coefficient among those who below the minimally adequate level of health. The SST measure takes value between 0 and 1, and a smaller value suggests a greater achievement of the minimally adequate level of health in a population.

Reflecting our discussion in chapter 4, table E.1 compares important properties of these two measures. Table E also comes with my suggestion of relative priorities of these theoretical considerations. Three desirable characteristics of poverty measures proposed by Sen are the most important properties. Next, one should look at the questions discussed in chapter 4. Finally, one can examine the same question for the inequality measure among those who are below the minimally adequate level of health.

Considering the first priority, both FGT and SST measures are on an equal footing. A difference between them begins to appear regarding the second priority. Sen suggests that the primary reason why the FGT measure is more widely used than the SST measure in poverty studies is the FGT's decomposability by subpopulation (Sen 1997, 180).[13] Is this decomposability also an attractive property in health inequity analysis? Note that decomposition by subgroup is different for inequality measure and poverty measures:

Additively decomposable inequality measure:[14]

$$I_{total} = I_{within\text{-}group} + I_{between\text{-}group}.$$

Additively decomposable poverty measure:

Table E.1
The FGT measure versus the SST measure

	FGT (a=2) Foster, Greer, Thorbecke	SST Sen, Shorrocks, Thon
Overall properties – the 1st priority		
Head-count	Yes	Yes
How many people are below the poverty line?		
Poverty gap	Yes, applied to everyone	Yes, applied to the poor only
What is the gap between the poor and the poverty line on average ...		
... *over all people?*		... *over the poor?*
Inequality among the poor	Yes, by the squared coefficient of variation	Yes, by the Gini coefficient
How is the income distributed among the poor?		
Overall properties – the 2nd priority		
Comparison	Anyone below the poverty line x the poverty line	Anyone below the poverty line x the poverty line
Aggregation	Weighted addition of difference (square)	Unweighted addtion of difference
Sensitivity to the mean	NA	NA
Sensitivity to the population size	Insensitive to the population size	Insensitive to the population size
Decomposition by subgroup	Additively decomposable	Not additively decomposable
Partial properties (with which inequality among the poor is measured) – the 3rd priority		
Comparison (among the poor)	Everyone x the mean income of the poor	Everyone x everyone
Aggregation	Weighted addition of health share	Weighted addition of health share
	Weighted addition of differences (square)	Unweighted addition of differences
Sensitivity to the mean	Scale invariant	Scale invariant
Sensitivity to the population size	Insensitive to the population size	Insensitive to the population size
Decomposition by subgroup	Additively decomposable	Non-additively decomposable

$$P_{total} = \frac{1}{N_{total}} \sum \left(P_{within\text{-}group} \cdot N_{group} \right).$$

Additively decomposable poverty measures only look at achievement of the threshold within groups but neglect the difference between groups. It is clear that the residual term of the Gini coefficient, which can be understood as overlap in decomposition of the Gini coefficient, does not allow additive decomposition of the SST measure. Indeed, to my knowledge, decomposition of the SST measure by subpopulation group has not been discussed in poverty literature.

Is an additively decomposable poverty measure desirable for analysis of health inequity from the perspective of health equity as satisfying the minimally adequate level of health? By analogy to Sen's argument for poverty analysis, the answer depends on the question we are asking, and how people below the threshold should be compared against the threshold (Sen 1997, 180–6). Let us see Sen's arguments in the health context.

There are two types of questions of likely interest in the analysis of health inequity with the idea of the minimally adequate level of health. The first is for which group health inequity is particularly bad. To answer this question, we would not need to use an additively decomposable measure; we can answer this question by examining health inequity in each group separately, even using a non-additively decomposable measure.

The second question is how much a given subpopulation contributes to overall health inequity. For this, we would need an additively decomposable measure. The desirability of an additively decomposable measure for health inequity analysis thus depends on the importance of the second question in health inequity analysis. While we can conduct a health inequity analysis for various reasons and with different interests, I think that in many cases we should be interested in the second question. Resources are limited to improve health equity, and it is useful to know how much difference it would make to overall health inequity if we could successfully bring everyone in a particular subpopulation to the minimally adequate level of health.

The second consideration Sen introduces in deciding whether it is desirable that a poverty measure be additively decomposable is theoretically interesting. He argues that the decision depends on how people below the threshold should be compared against the threshold. Should they be compared absolutely, that is, is what matters only the distance between a person's (health) level and the threshold? In this case, an additively decomposable measure is a good choice. Or should they be compared relatively, that is, does it also matter how other people fare in addition to the distance between a person's level and the threshold? This idea goes against the construction of an additively decomposable measure, and one should not choose an additively decomposable measure to reflect this idea. With the existence of the threshold, as Sen says for poverty measures, comparison of people from the perspective of health equity as satisfying the minimally adequate level of health is less relative than one in other perspectives on health equity. In the idea of the minimally adequate level of health, it seems logical that only the distance between a person's health level and the threshold matters. Therefore, here again an additively decomposable poverty measure appears to be desirable for health inequity analysis with the idea of minimally adequate level of health.

Among these theoretical considerations, the other difference between the FGT and SST measures is aggregation. The FGT measure uses weighted addition of differences while the SST measure uses unweighted addition of differences. In chapter 4, I argued that no weight should be attached to differences. Thus, in terms of aggregation, the SST measure appears to be a better choice than the FGT measure. However, I consider the importance of additive decomposability as more important than that of aggregation, and I rate the FGT measure more favourably than the SST measure. Although one could go on to examine more differences and desirable properties (for example, ones categorized in the third priority considerations), their importance is less than the properties we have already discussed. I therefore conclude that enough justification has been made for the FGT.

E.3. Subgroup Decomposition of the FGT Measure

The FTG measure is defined as[15]

$$P_\alpha = \frac{1}{N} \sum_{i=1}^{n} \left(\frac{z - y_i}{z} \right)^\alpha,$$

where $y = (y_1, y_1, ..., y_N)$ is a vector of health in increasing order, z is the threshold line, $z - y_i$ is the health shortfalls of the ith individual, N is the total population, and n is the total number of those who below the threshold. Suppose we have subgroups $j = 1, 2, ..., m$. Foster, Greer, and

Thorbecke show subgroup decomposition of the FGT measure is possible in the following way:

$$P_\alpha = \sum_{j=1}^{m} \frac{N_j}{N} \cdot P_\alpha^j,$$

where N_j is the total population of subgroup j, P_α^j is the FGT measure for the subgroup j. The total FGT measure is additively decomposable with population share weights.[16]

E.4. Statistical Inference for the FGT Measure

I use the method proposed by Jolliffe and Semykina to draw a statistical inference for the FGT measure (1999). Jolliffe and Semykina suggest that additive decomposability of the FGT measure provides a convenient way to obtain standard errors of the FGT measure. As mentioned in section E.2, the FGT measure can be decomposed as follows:

$$P_\alpha = \sum_{j=1}^{m} \frac{N_j}{N} \cdot P_\alpha^j,$$

where N_j is the total population of subgroup j, P_α^j is the FGT measure for the subgroup j. If each observation in data is considered as a subgroup, the total FGT (P_α), is the mean of observation-specific estimates of the FGT (P_α^j). Accounting for the complex survey design of the NHIS, this mean is estimated with appropriate weights, and its standard error by linearization method (first-order Taylor expansion) (StataCorp 1999a, 4:51–72).

Appendix F:
Adjustment of Household Income for Family Size and Structure

Depending on family size and structure, the value of the same household income would be different. Household income, therefore, should be adjusted for family size and structure. The NHIS, however, does not provide household income as the exact amount, which makes this adjustment difficult. Table F.1 presents selected results of the mean HALex and the Gini coefficient by income group stratified by family size for 1995. For families up to five members, the relationship between income and the mean HALex or the Gini coefficient is stable: we observe the same graded relationship as for no stratification by family size. For families with more than six members, on the other hand, this relationship does not always hold. This suggests that if table 6.6 were adjusted for the family size, we would observe a weaker relationship between income and the mean HALex or the Gini coefficient than is now presented in table 6.6.

Table F.1
The mean HALex and the Gini coefficient in 1995 by income stratified by family size

	Household income				
	<$15,000	$15,000–$24,999	$25,000–$34,999	$35,000–$49,999	$50,000+
Mean HALex					
Family size	0.73	0.78	0.83	0.88	0.90
3	0.82	0.84	0.88	0.89	0.92
5	0.85	0.87	0.90	0.91	0.94
7	0.85	0.86	0.90	0.90	0.90
9+	0.87	0.83	0.87	0.88	0.93
Gini coefficient					
Family size					
3	0.127	0.115	0.086	0.076	0.061
5	0.099	0.089	0.073	0.060	0.049
7	0.099	0.096	0.075	0.077	0.074
9+	0.085	0.108	0.090	0.088	0.059

Notes

1. Introduction

1 See 'inequality' and 'unequal' in *The American Heritage Dictionary* (Pickett et al. 2000). For the precise definition of inequality used in this book, see section 1.4.

2 See an accessible and insightful discussion on 'equality of what?' by Sen (1992, 12–30).

3 In recent years, for example, health inequality has been a popular theme topic for academic journals and conferences in a variety of disciplines. Special theme issues include 'Health inequalities in modern societies and beyond,' *Social Science and Medicine* 44(6), 1997, 'Social and economic disparities in health,' *Milbank Quarterly* 76(3), 1998, and 'Inequalities in health,' *Bulletin of the World Health Organization* 78(1), 2000. Academic conferences that focused on health inequality include biannual conferences of the International Society for Equity in Health (ISEqH) and the 128th annual meeting of the American Public Health Association in 2000. See Machinko and Starfield (2002) for a useful annotated bibliography of health inequality research between 1980 and 2001.

4 Marmot (2001) provides a brief history of *The Black Report* and its impact.

5 There is a large literature on inequalities in health care by race or ethnicity (for example, Freeman and Payne 2000; Mayberry, Mili, and Ofili 2000; Smedley, Stith, and Nelson 2002; Weinick and Zuvekas 2000) and inequalities in health by race or ethnicity (for example, Keppel, Pearcy, and Wagener 2002; Thomas 2001). Feinstein (1993) and Raphael (2000) provide reviews of health inequality in the U.S.

6 O'Neil (2003) gives general discussion on measurements and accountability.

7 As this example illustrates, supporters of the right to health may argue that one should look at the entire health distribution across individuals. In

chapter 2, I introduce another view, the right to the minimally adequate level of health. Supporters of this view would only look at the distribution of health across individuals below a threshold.

8 This view, for example, is proposed by Starfield (2001) and Braveman and Gruskin (2003a).

9 HRQL is a measurement of health status, mapping all possible health states between dead (zero) and full health (one). A larger value indicates a better state of health. The Gini coefficient is a measurement expressing the degree of health inequality. Zero indicates perfect equality, and one most unequal. The research results introduced here are from Asada and Ohkusa (2004). For related discussion, see section 6.2 in chapter 6.

10 See, on this point, Brock (2000), Daniels, Kennedy, and Kawachi (2000), Peter and Evans (2001), Powers and Faden (2000), and Wikler (1997).

11 See Brock (2000), Daniels, Kennedy, and Kawachi (2000), Peter and Evans (2001), Powers and Faden (2000), and Marchand, Wikler, and Landesman (1998).

12 See Williams and Cookson (2000), Culyer (2001), and Bommier and Stecklov (2002) for pioneering work by economists on the moral implications of health inequality.

13 See *Tackling Health Inequalities: A Programme for Action* (UK Department of Health 2003, 7).

14 See Braveman and Tarimo (2002) for health inequality in developed countries. For the persistent health inequality after establishment of a universal health care system in the UK and Canada, see Black (1982) and Badgley (1991). For health inequality in Scandinavian countries, see Lahelma, et al. (2002). For health inequality in Japan, see Asada and Ohkusa (2004) and Shibuya, Hashimoto, and Yano (2002).

15 An excellent overview of how the relationship between health and socio-economic status has been studied can be found in Robert and House (2000). Regarding age and the relationship between SES and health, see House et al. (1990). Regarding sex, see Mustard and Etches (2003). Regarding various measurements of health, see Adler et al. (1993).

16 The quote is from Adler et al. (1993, 3143). For the resource argument, see Feinstein (1993). For the information argument, see Adler et al. (1993). For the psychological argument, see Adler et al. (1994).

17 For recent overview of income inequality research, see, for example, Kawachi, Kennedy, and Wilkinson (1999), Lynch et al. (2004a), Lynch et al. (2004b), Ross (2004), Subramanian and Kawachi (2004), Wagstaff and van Doorslaer (2000), and Wilkinson and Pickett (2006).

18 For a collection of important papers on social cohesion and social capital,

see the section entitled 'Social Cohesion and Health' in Kawachi, Kennedy, and Wilkinson (1999, 161–277).

19 Visit *The World Health Report* homepage http://www.who.int/whr/en/ for general information. For a general critique of *The World Health Report 2000* (World Health Organization 2000a), see the editorials of the medical journals, the *Lancet* (*Why rank countries* 2001) and the *British Medical Journal* (McKee 2001), and papers by Almeida et al. (2001), Navarro (2002), and Williams (2001).

20 Throughout the book, I mean the WHO health inequality index by the health inequality measure proposed by Gakidou, Murray, and Frenk for *The World Health Report 2000* (Gakidou, Murray, and Frenk 2000; Murray, Gakidou, and Frenk 1999). Although the order of the authorship differs in different papers, for consistency I refer to these researchers as Gakidou, Murray, and Frenk.

21 Papers critiquing the WHO's health inequality measure include Asada and Hedemann (2002), Braveman, Krieger, and Lynch (2000), Braveman, Starfield, and Geiger (2001), Hausman, Asada, and Hedemann (2002), Leon, Walt, and Gilson (2001), Szwarcwald (2002), and Wolfson and Rowe (2001).

22 Temkin refers to this third step as 'when is one situation worse than another regarding inequality?' (1993, 3).

23 See, for example, Braveman (2006) for various definitions of these terms proposed in health sciences literature.

24 Cater-Pokras and Baquet (2002) provide a useful summary of a diverse use of 'disparity,' a popular term in the U.S.

25 Suppose that genocide occurred in a population. Everyone in this population is dead, thus health (that is, death, in this example) is equally distributed in this population. Despite the equal distribution of a health state, the moral objection is obvious. It is therefore better to state that some health *distributions* are of moral concern than that some health *inequalities* are of moral concern. Still, it is perhaps correct to assume that there are more inequitable inequalities than inequitable equalities, and under this assumption, in the following discussion, I sometimes speak of health *inequalities* as moral concerns.

26 Different people use the term 'egalitarianism' differently. Some take the meaning of egalitarianism literally as anyone seeking (whatever kind of) equality and include utilitarianism as a form of egalitarianism in the understanding that every person is counted equally in the utilitarian perspective. Even in this use of the term, I believe the classification of distribution-insensitive ethical and moral interest in health inequality and distribution-sensitive interest still stands.

27 Throughout this book, by 'social justice' I literally mean 'justice in society.' Some scholars limit 'social justice' to mean no systematic oppression of social groups. In this view, the unit of analysis of social justice must be the group (Feminist Health Care Ethics Research Network et al. 1998; Young 1990). I take the meaning of social justice more broadly, and in my usage, social justice does not presume a particular unit of analysis.

28 All quotes of Jefferson in this paragraph are from Jefferson (1787).

29 In philosophical discussion of equality, philosophers talk about ethical concerns regarding equality, which is, in my terminology, equity. In the philosophy literature, however, they are usually referred to as arguments on equality, not equity, and I follow this custom here.

30 In this paragraph, I follow an excellent summary of philosophical discussion on equality in Hausman and McPherson (2006, chapter 11). For resourcist views, see Dworkin (1981b) and Rawls (1971). For welfarist views, see Dworkin (1981a). For the view of opportunities for welfare, see Arneson (1989). For the capability approach, see Nussbaum (2000) and Sen (1992).

31 Other scholars, however, do not believe that health should be included in the list of goods whose distribution is of moral interest. For example, Dworkin does not include health or health care in his list of resources to be equalized. In his view, we should equalize income (and other resources) so people can buy health insurance according to their life plans (Dworkin 1981b; Marchand, Wikler, and Landesman 1998).

2. Which Health Distributions Are Inequitable?

1 See Williams and Cookson (2000) for a review of how philosophical theories of distributive justice can apply to welfare economics.

2 One exception where prioritarians and egalitarians make different judgments is under uncertainty. See Broome (n.d.) and Fleurbaey (n.d. a).

3 See the discussion on aggregation in chapter 4, section 4.4 for a possible measurement approach that prioritarians might take.

4 Unless, of course, we kill all the sick. Although this is a possibility to realize health equality, I do not treat this option seriously, as it is obviously morally objectionable.

5 Or, more precisely, chance acquisition *starts* at the very beginning of life for genetics given the complex interactions between genes and environments.

6 See Kekes (1997) for a philosophical discussion of whether inequality in life expectancy between men and women is inequitable and Tsuchiya and

Williams (2005) for an examination of the same question from the perspective of 'fair innings.'

7 For example, see Cappelen and Norheim (2005; 2006), Fleurbaey (n.d. b), Gakidou, Murray, and Frenk (2000), Van de Vathorst and Alvarez-Dardet (2000), and Wikler (2004).

8 Dan Brock argues that if health inequalities caused by factors within social control are really inequitable, given that health care is only a partial determinant of such health inequalities, we must extend our interest in inequity in health care to inequity in health (2000).

9 Who the poor are is itself an interesting question. Gwatkin notes that the World Bank has changed its definition of the poor; according to the new definition, health is considered to be a component of poverty rather than its determinant (2000). Consequently, the World Bank's attention to the health of the poor, in the old definition, should be the health of the poor, however defined, but in the new definition, could be the health of the sick (Wagstaff 2001).

10 The problem discussed here may only be methodological; that is, the theory is sound, but we do not know how to implement it. However, as we discuss later, genetics as a determinant of health implies a theoretical difficulty in this perspective on health equity.

11 A qualification applies as to how men's life years are prolonged. Suppose that a special diet can extend the human lifespan. With this special diet, men can extend their life years and catch up with women's. But is it acceptable to provide this special diet to men only? A further justification is necessary to establish the moral acceptability of filling the gap in life years between men and women.

12 Of course, as discussed, it is possible to combine this perspective with a certain view of health inequality and biological variation. It might then judge that health inequality caused by sex is not inequitable.

13 See, for example, Braveman, Krieger, and Lynch (2000) and Braveman, Starfield, and Geiger (2001).

14 The idea of the minimally adequate level of health can also be seen as a variant of the argument of a right to health (for example, Braveman and Gruskin 2003b; Griffin n.d.; Mann 1997). Braveman and Gruskin state that the right to health in the international human rights treaties and the WHO constitution means 'the highest attainable standard of health' and propose to operationalize it as the 'standard of health enjoyed by the most socially advantaged group within a society' (2003b, 255). For the argument of a right to health to be of any importance, one must start by examining whether any right to health can be justified, and if so, what it exactly is.

For this reason, a general philosophical discussion of equality and justice is necessary prior to arguing a right to health (Daniels 1985, 4–9), and this is exactly what I am trying to do here.

15 We must also examine whether reproduction should even be included in the opportunity at all. The inclusion of reproduction requires an expansive notion of opportunity.

16 To examine this question, we must first closely look at health. When we do so in chapter 3, it will become clear that the normal species functioning view and the capability approach would define the minimum level of health differently. I will then come back to the question of the feasibility of defining the minimum level of health.

17 It is unclear whether we should consider equity perspectives that do not take care of the cost issue as incomplete. The question of whether equity should always be examined with other ideals is yet to obtain a consensus (Temkin 1993, 7; Williams 1997a, 346). For further discussion, see chapter 4.

18 This is one of the distinct characteristics of health distribution as opposed to income distribution.

19 Similar to the views introduced in this section, an ecosocial perspective suggests that health inequality can be considered as an indicator of vulnerability underlying a population (Galea, Ahern, and Karpati 2005; Levins and Lopez 1999). According to this perspective, stressors affect more vulnerable human populations with greater severity than they do less vulnerable populations and lead to greater variability in health in these populations. This view is biological rather than egalitarian, yet it connects with the views introduced in this section in terms of our judgment on the degree of health inequality.

3. What Measurement Choices Must Be Faced to Measure Health Inequity?

1 Cutting-edge health status measures often controversially vary in various aspects. Williams and Cookson think that different perspectives on health equity might favour particular types of health status measures (2000). Future work is necessary on this point.

2 In chapter 2, we discussed the uncertainty over whether health should be considered as capability or functioning in Sen's version of the capability approach. Assuming that Sen's version regards health as a capability, it is not obvious whether the capability approach, either Nussbaum's or Sen's, focuses on capacity or performance in the ICF classification. Nussbaum talks about universal values in capabilities (2000, chap. 1), but both ver-

sions are concerned about *equivalent* rather than *equal* capability. Thus, both versions would seek some environmental adjustments in their considerations for capability.

3 Economists might say that health as functionality, discussed in this section, can be best understood as a non-final commodity. 'Final commodities' in economics are commodities destined for final consumption, and 'non-final commodities' are commodities that flow into intermediate consumption for further processing.

4 This argument may sound obvious to philosophers, and it should be to anyone. But to empirical analysts, in the pure statistical sense, the more inequality a distribution exhibits, the more interesting it appears. Thus, a reminder is necessary as to why we are here interested in health inequality.

5 Imagine a society in which everyone's level of health is above the minimally adequate level, but the stature of people belonging to a certain ethnic group is below this level. These people are as healthy as anyone else but extremely short, much below the minimally adequate stature, due to a certain gene passed onto this ethnic group for generations. The capability approach must say that health is not equitably distributed in this society. However, given that the ancestral genetic factor is solely responsible for the inequitable health distribution in this society, this conclusion seems to be absurd. Future work is necessary to investigate whether the capability approach is truly free from any causal relationship.

6 Genetic endowment in the Evans-Stoddart model can be considered a chance determinant. In chapter 2, though, we discussed how complicated it is to characterize genetics as a determinant of health, which raises another issue later in this section.

7 Sen's framework for thinking about health equity (2002b) can be seen as an expansion of figure 3.3. Sen believes that we should consider a complex notion of health equity as complex. Accordingly, he suggests that, in addition to components in figure 3.3, we must also think of social arrangements of other goods (for example, income and education), and how health is produced from determinants to expectation and outcomes.

8 For example, Dworkin (1981b), Daniels, Kennedy, and Kawachi (2000).

9 See Feeny et al. (1995), Salomon et al. (2003), Ware et al. (1981), and the World Health Organization (2001).

10 Health-related quality of life (HRQL) scores are, as shown in table 3.2, numerical values assigned to different health states based on people's preferences.

11 The answer to the question of which level of functionality and general symptoms health status measures should assess ultimately depends on what

it is about health that we wish to measure. I believe the view of health as a multi-purpose resource is a fundamental value that drives us to seek health equity, but there may be other views, for example, the primary reason why we care about health inequity is it causes suffering. The view of Reidpath, Allotey, and their colleagues appears to be compatible with this view (Allotey et al. 2003; Reidpath et al. 2003). They argue that the Disability-Adjusted Life Year (DALY) should measure the burden of disease 'as it truly occurs' (Reidpath et al. 2003, 354). In this view, DALY should include not only medical technologies and non-human aids but also human assistance and environmental factors.

12 The discussion in the following paragraph can be extended to any self-perceived health, that is, asking people to assess their health state as opposed to using examinations or expert opinions. Sen calls self-perceived health in this inclusive sense the 'internal' views, and the other, 'external' views (2002a, 860). He warns against the recent blind reliance on the internal views in measuring health.

13 Not in the health equity context, but health care resource allocation context, many scholars agree, albeit with different reasons, that it is morally acceptable to prioritize the young over the old when they have the same health state. See, for example, Anand (2005), Brouwer, van Exel, and Stolk (2005), Callahan (1987), Tsuchiya (2000), Veatch (1988), and Williams (1997a).

14 McKerlie opposes this view in the context of general equality or justice (1992; 1997; 2002). He believes that being old cannot itself justify being sick, poor, and miserable, and irrespective of age, we should be concerned about who is the worst-off at a particular time. I think that this claim may stand in thinking of justice in general but probably not in the health context. As we have discussed, the biological process of ageing has a strong influence on how much health one is likely to obtain, and this circumstance is shared by all humans. We might think that well-being should not be determined by age, but it seems reasonable to think that the contribution of health to well-being declines in old age.

15 For rare examples of measuring health inequality across individuals apart from the work by Gakidou, Murray, and Frenk for the WHO, see Illsley and Le Grand (1987), Le Grand (1987), Pradhan, Sahn, and Younger (2003), and Silber (1982). For the proposal to measure health inequality across individuals by Gakidou, Murray, and Frenk, see Gakidou, Murray, and Frenk (2000) and Murray, Gakidou, and Frenk (1999). Papers critiquing this proposal include Almeida et al. (2001), Asada and Hedemann (2002), Braveman (2001), Braveman, Krieger, and Lynch (2000), Brave-

man, Starfield, and Geiger (2001), Hausman, Asada, and Hedemann (2002), Szwarcwald (2002), Ugá et al. (2001), and Wolfson and Rowe (2001).

16 For an extended discussion on whether health inequality across individuals is of moral concern, see Asada (2006) and Hausman (2007).

17 See Almeida et al. (2001), Anand (2002), Braveman (2001), Braveman, Krieger, and Lynch (2000), and Braveman, Starfield, and Geiger (2001).

18 For excellent overviews of measuring health, see, for example, Field and Gold (1998), Gold, Stevenson, and Fryback (2002), and Murray et al. (2002).

4. How Can a Health Distribution Be Summarized into One Number?

1 In his review of inequality measurements, Philip Coulter distinguishes inequality measures from inequity measures (1989). He sees that in measuring inequity, one must define an independent, standard distribution, and the 'extent of inequity characterizing a distribution is measured with respect to its divergence from some other distribution among the components of the same system' (Coulter 1989, 161). I suspect that in this approach to measuring inequity, what is inequitable or equitable has not been sorted out in the distribution; the distribution of interest contains inequity information of interest and more. In my approach, and presumably the approach in income inequality measurement, the distribution of interest only contains inequity information of interest through defining inequity and choosing measurement strategies before drawing the distribution.

2 This includes measuring health distribution for non-ethical reasons. In such a case, answers to these distinct questions would not reflect equity questions. But distinct questions do arise and must be answered if one wants to summarize health distribution into one number.

3 What should we do when there are so many inequality measures that we want to compare? The intersection approach may not be practical. Economists suggest that rather than comparing all possible inequality measures, we should first come up with inequality measures that satisfy certain properties and then see how they rank distributions. It turns out that for inequality measures that satisfy properties of symmetry (inequality measures only measure the distributional good of focus, for example, income or health, irrespective of any other characteristics of individuals, for example, personality), scale invariance, insensitivity to population replication, and the Pigou-Dalton condition (regressive transfer increases

inequality while progressive transfer decreases inequality) can be compared by using the Lorenz Curve. This approach is called Lorenz Dominance (Coulter 1989, 22–4; Litchfield 1999; Sen 1997, 142–5). The useful-
ness of this approach obviously depends on whether we wish to consider
these four properties as attractive. As I argue in this chapter, I think some
of these properties may not be attractive in measuring health inequality.

4 Here my points regarding the intersection approach refer specifically to
applying it to the health context. See Temkin (1993, 141–7) for problems
of the intersection approach in general.

5 In economic thinking of population health production, everything
appears to be reduced either to equity or efficiency. Harming the healthy,
for example, is an efficiency issue, but in philosophy it may be categorized
under a different ideal, 'Do no harm.'

6 See, for example, Bleichrodt and van Doorslaer (2006), Dolan and Olsen
(2001), Lindholm and Rosen (1998), Olsen (1997), Silber (1982),
Wagstaff (2002a), and Williams (1997b).

7 See Atkinson (1970, 251), Sen (1997, 36–7), and Temkin (Temkin 1993,
chap. 6).

8 For the axiomatic approach, see, for example, Cowell (1995; 2000),
Kakwani (1980), Litchfield (1999), and Sen (1997). For the axiomatic
approach specifically in the health context, see Anand et al. (2001), Fleurbaey (n.d. b), Harper and Lynch (2005), Keppel, Pearcy, and Klein
(2004), Keppel et al. (2005), Levy, Chemerynski, and Tuchmann (2006),
Mackenbach and Kunst (1997), Manor, Matthews, and Power (1997), and
Wagstaff, Paci, and van Doorslaer (1991).

9 For income inequality research, see Amiel and Cowell (1992; 1998) and
Harrison and Seidl (1994). For health inequality research, see Dolan and
Shaw (2001) and Gakidou, Murray, and Frenk (2001).

10 I will mention this more specifically with the example of fig. 4.5a.

11 For example, see Hosseinpoor et al. (2005), Humphries and van Doorslaer
(2000), Koolman and van Doorslaer (2004), and van Doorslaer and
Koolman (2004).

12 See Almeida et al. (2001), Asada and Henemann (2002), Braveman
(2001), Braveman, Krieger, and Lynch (2000), Braveman, Starfield,
and Geiger (2001), Hausman, Asada, and Hedemann. (2002),
Gakidou, Murray, and Frenk (2000), Murray, Gakidou, and Frenk (1999;
2000), Szwarcwald (2002), Ugá et al. (2001), and Wolfson and Rowe
(2001).

13 For a review of inequality measures in the health context, see Anand et al.
(2001), Carr-Hill and Chalmers-Dixon (2005), Harper and Lynch (2005),
Mackenbach and Kunst (1997), Manor, Matthews, and Power (1997),

Regidor (2004a; 2004b), and Wagstaff, Paci, and van Doorslaer (1991). For a review of inequality measures in general, see, for example, Coulter (1989) and Sen (1997).

14 Or, using John Broome's terminology, a 'claim' (1989).

15 Hilary Graham's examination of health inequality policy documents in the UK from 1997 to 2003 suggests that policy documents are not necessarily always clear about which comparison concept they opt for (2004). She points out that these UK policy documents appear to focus either on the worst-off ('remedying health disadvantages'), the worst-off in relation to the best-off ('narrowing health gaps'), or all social groups ('reducing health gradients') (Graham 2004, 115).

16 The WHO health inequality index type of measurement is

$\frac{1}{2} \sum_{i=1}^{n} \sum_{j=1}^{n} \frac{|y_i - y_j|^\alpha}{n^2 \mu^\beta}$, where the population of interest holds n people, y_i is

the health of individual i, y_j is the health of individual j, the average level of health in the population is μ, and $\alpha = 3$ and $\beta = 0.56$. When $\alpha = 1$ and $\beta = 1$, this measure is equivalent to the Gini coefficient.

17 Both the extended Concentration Index and Gini coefficient can be

expressed as $1 - \dfrac{\sum_{i=1}^{n} \left(R_i^\nu - (R_i - 1)^\nu \right) y_i}{n^\nu \mu}$, where the population of interest

holds n people, y_i is the health of individual i, the average level of health in the population is μ, and R_i is the relative rank of the individual i, 1 suggesting the best rank. The ranking is in terms of socio-economic status for the Concentration Index and health for the Gini coefficient. When $\nu = 2$, this measure becomes the standard Concentration Index or the Gini coefficient (Bleichrodt and van Doorslaer 2006; Wagstaff 2002a).

18 In addition to the basic reasoning introduced here, which should apply to any population, when measuring individual health in a very healthy population we might wish to 'discount' the health of the people at the higher end of the distribution. While it is fully understandable that someone may have a complaint against the very healthiest person from the perspective of individuals, we might want to question whether we should count this complaint fully at the policy level. Perhaps the very healthiest person in a population is a mystery case of human health many of whose factors are beyond our understanding. Good timing and lots of luck alone may greatly account for health. For this reason, we may not want to count complaints against the healthiest person as much as against less healthy people. And if this is true, then we may count complaints against the second healthiest person a little less. This can go on and on, and it is not

~~clear from what health level we might want to employ this idea.~~ Yet it is clear that, according to this idea, we would wish to apply some sort of asymmetric weighting.

19 Inequality measures using parameters α and v can be different in terms of the sensitivity to the mean and the scale within which inequality measures take values. Following the expressions already introduced above, the WHO health inequality index type of measurement can be expressed as

as $W' = \dfrac{1}{2} \displaystyle\sum_{i=1}^{n} \sum_{j=1}^{n} \dfrac{|y_i - y_j|^{\alpha}}{n^2 \mu}$, and the extended Gini coefficient,

$EG = 1 - \dfrac{\displaystyle\sum_{i=1}^{n} \left(R_i^{\,v} - (R_i - 1)^{v} \right) y_i}{n^{v} \mu}$ When $\alpha = 1$ and $v = 2$, $W' = EG$ and these

measures are the standard Gini coefficient. Selecting values for α and v, W' and EG can express similar concerns for the sicker persons and larger differences between health (Norheim 2006). However, the sensitivity to the mean of these measures can vary. Whatever value v takes, EG is always scale invariant. On the other hand, when $\alpha = 1$ W' is scale invariant but when $\alpha > 1$, W' expresses intermediate inequality. The difference in the sensitivity to the mean between these measures comes from n^{v} in the denominator of EG and n^2 in the denominator of W'. This observation suggests that different questions (aggregation, sensitivity to the mean, and sensitivity to the population size) addressed separately in this book eventually need to be discussed together. Another difference between W' and EG is that whatever value v takes, EG always takes values between zero and one, while using a greater value of α, W' can take values greater than one. While W' may not need to be confined between zero and one, the zero-one unit does provide convenient comparability of inequalities. For a discussion on the sensitivity to the mean and the sensitivity to the population size, see the following sections in this chapter. For an example of W' taking greater values than one, see appendix B1.

20 I use the term 'mean' as a representative level of the overall population health. Discussion in this section is not a statistical question of which 'central tendency' measures – mean, median, or mode – can best describe the population's overall health. While this is an interesting question in health inequality measurement, I assume that the mean is a good central tendency measure in this book.

21 See, for example, Atkinson (1970, 251), Clarke et al. (2002), Mackenbach and Kunst (1997), Sen (1997, 36–7), Temkin (1993, chap. 6), and Wagstaff, Paci, and van Doorslaer (1991).

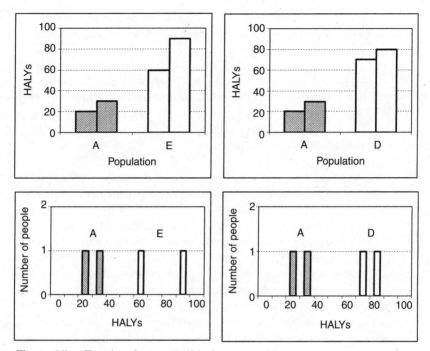

Figure 4.5a   Framing due to graphical presentation

22 Note that graphical presentation of health inequality is likely to frame our thinking of inequality. Look at figure 4.5a, in which Population A, E, and D from figure 4.5 are presented in two different ways. In this book I will not further discuss a possibility of framing due to graphical presentation, but this is an important issue for the future.

23 For example, Cowell (2000) uses 'compromise inequality,' and Bossert and Pfingsten (1990), Dutta and Esteban (1991), Rio and Ruiz-Castillo (2000), and Seidl and Pfingsten (1997) use 'intermediate inequality.'

24 Literature on health inequality measurement has often asked how one should perceive differences – absolutely or relatively – rather than whether health inequality measurement should be sensitive to the population's mean level (for example, Anand et al. 2001; Low and Low 2006; Lynch et al. 2006; Mustard and Etches 2003). Yet, as I explain in this section, these two questions are phrasing the same question differently.

25 Discussing population prevention strategies rather than health inequality, Geoffrey Rose advocates absolute risks for their policy relevance: 'Relative

risk is not what decision-taking requires, for doubling a trivial risk is still trivial but doubling a common risk is alarming. "Relative risk" is only for researchers; decisions call for absolute measures' (1992, 19).

26 For example, comparing situations such as Population A, B, and D, health sciences researchers have pointed out that inequality measures looking at differences relatively tend to give us a large degree of inequality at a very low value (Anand et al. 2001). To my knowledge, there is little discussion among health sciences researchers as to whether we should consider this property favourable or problematic in measuring health inequality, and for what reasons.

27 Williams and Cookson (2000) agree with me on this point, and their discussion on the sensitivity to the population size is as exploratory as this section.

28 There is an exceptional case. Suppose that in Population A, Group 1 exhibits a lower level of health than Group 2, and in Population B, Group 2 exhibits a lower level of health than Group 1. If inequalities in Population A and B were the exact mirror image, the total population, in which A and B were united, would have perfect equality (inequality between Population A and B would be zero, and inequalities within A and B would cancel out). While this could occur, it would be an exceptional case of uniting two populations. Thus, I assume that the claim supported by economists is still valid that it is *generally* believed that inequality of the total population is at least as great as or worse than inequality of subpopulations.

29 See Almeida et al. (2001), Asada and Hedemann (2002), Braveman (2001), Braveman, Krieger, and Lynch (2000), Hausman, Asada, and Hedemann (2002), and Leon, Walt, and Gilson (2001).

30 I adopted most of the discussion in the first two paragraphs from Sen's explanation on subgroup consistency (1997, 149–63).

31 See, for example, Dagum (1997), Lambert and Aronson (1993), Warner (2001), Yitzhaki (1994), and Yitzhaki and Lerman (1991). Wagstaff and van Doorslaer explain subgroup decomposition of the Gini coefficient in the context of 'overall versus socioeconomic health inequality' (2004, 297) and in relation to the Concentration Index.

32 A further issue arises when we think of subgroup decomposition and the subgroup size together. The degree of stratification is obviously dependent on the subgroup size. Whether we wish to control the subgroup size in examining the degree of stratification is a moot point, but for either decision, an index of stratification is available (Yitzhaki and Lerman 1991).

33 As I mentioned at the outset, this chapter has used the term 'inequality

measures' rather than 'inequity measures' following the customary use of terminology in the literature. Chapters 2 and 3 help in the extraction of health inequity information on which to focus, and this chapter assists in summarizing that information into one number. Thus, health inequality measures in this chapter are, in a precise sense, health inequity measures.

5. Bridging Concepts and Analysis

1 Moreover, death represents an extreme score in health status measures, including the HALex. Analysis of a distribution is likely to be sensitive to an extreme value, thus, inclusion of the dead is also meaningful in this regard.

2 For example, see Gakidou and King (2002), Keppel, Pearcy, and Wagener (2002), van Doorslaer and Koolman (2004), and the World Health Organization (2000a).

3 As mentioned in the beginning of chapter 4, the distinction between inequality and inequity is not usually made in the field of measurement of a distribution. Inequality measures can be used for summarizing a distribution carrying any information, including inequity information. In the following, I use the terms 'inequality measures' and 'inequity measures' interchangeably, when inequality measures summarize inequity information.

4 The following description of the NHIS is summarized from *Design and Estimation for the National Health Interview Survey, 1985–94* and *1995–2004* (Botman et al. 2000; Massey et al. 1989).

5 For a useful introduction on this issue, see, for example, Froberg and Kane (1989a; 1989b; 1989c; 1989d) and Fryback (1998).

6 Because both information on activity limitation and self-perceived health is collected by a self-report of survey respondents, questions remain as to how much of the HALex is objective health and how much is influenced by the expectation of survey respondents. Studies suggest that the health status assessed by medical equipment or health professionals and the health status assessed by an individual do not always agree with each other (Sen 2002a). Whose assessment of health we should use in health inequity analysis is an important question, and this is an area where the development of health inequity measurement and that of health status measurement must proceed together.

7 See Greenacre (1992; 2002) for a detailed explanation of correspondence analysis.

8 Drummond et al. (1997) gives a detailed explanation of multi-attribute

utility theory, and technical notes of the YHL (Erickson, Wilson, and Shannon 1995) provide further detail of the HALex construction.

9 For decomposition of the Gini coefficient, see, for example, Lambert and Aronson (1993), Pyatt (1976), Wagstaff and van Doorslaer (2004), Yao (1999), Yitzhaki (1994), and Yitzhaki and Lerman (1991). Regarding statistical inference of the Gini coefficient, see, for example, Karagiannis and Kovacevic (2000), Mills and Zandvakili (1997), Ogwang (2000), and Zheng (2001).

10 See Jolliffe and Krushelnytskyy (1999), McCarthy and Snowden (1985), and Sitter (1992).

11 An empirical study by Ferrer and Palmer (2004) suggests that investigation of inequality within groups and overlap between groups would indeed be interesting. Using a nationally representative sample of about 50,000 adults in the U.S. in 1996, they showed that the health of the healthiest 25% within the top income quintile group was almost the same as the health of the healthiest 25% within the bottom income quintile group. Differences in health between the five income groups mostly came from how sick the sicker members were within each income group.

12 For the Foster-Greer-Thorbecke (FGT) measure, see Foster, Greer, and Thorbecke (1984). For the Sen-Shorrocks-Thon (SST) measure, see Sen (1976), Shorrocks (1995), and Thon (1979; 1983).

13 For example, see Howes and Lanjouw (1998) and Osberg and Xu (1999; 2000).

14 Recall also that, unlike the whole-life approach, the life-stage approach does not take death into account. The dead imputation I use in analyses in part 2 is one way to incorporate death into the life-stage approach. See section 3.3 of chapter 3.

15 This raises a couple of questions. First, is women's health status objectively lower than men's? Or do women perceive their health status as lower than men's though the objective health status may be similar between women and men? One problem with the HALex is that activity limitation is also self-reported, thus, the distribution of activity limitation does not really show the objective picture of health status measured, for example, by medical equipment. Besides, even if we discovered that women perceive the same, objective health conditions lower than men, we must further ask if such perception should be treated as a health problem. This same question can be raised for any other variables, that is, health perception by socio-economic status, racial/ethnic groups, or geographic location. Another question relates to the HALex construction. How much of the HALex is influenced by self-perceived health? If activity limitation does

not in an important way contribute to the HALex, the HALex score could be constructed only from self-perceived health data, which are ubiquitous in health surveys.

6. Did Health Equity Improve in the United States between 1990 and 1995?

1 This study only compares health inequity in 1990 and 1995, thus, strictly speaking, it does not provide information of a *trend*. Routine collection of health inequity every year will enable a richer assessment of health inequity in the future.

2 The variance (V) is defined as $V = \sum_{i=1}^{n} \frac{(\mu - y_i)^2}{n}$; where the population of interest has n people, each of them possesses the health level y, and the average level of health in the population is μ. In the following cases where the Gini coefficient and the variance do not agree in terms of whether health inequality in 1990 and 1995 were different: 45–64 years old for both sexes, 65+ years old among men, and 0–14 and 45–64 years old among women in the living and the dead population, and 65+ years old among women in the living population. In other cases, the difference between them is how much difference exists between 1990 and 1995.

3 The dead imputed do have information on sex. But for consistency, I use only the living population for the decomposition by sex.

4 See Kawachi, Daniels, and Robinson (2005) for the discussion of why health inequities by race and socio-economic status are important, and why neither can substitute the other.

5 Both in 1990 and 1995, death rates were higher among Blacks than Whites or other races. Death rates per 100,000 persons adjusted for the U.S. population in 1940 are, for Blacks, 787.2 in 1990 and 766.4 in 1995; for Whites, 492.2 in 1990 and 476.6 in 1995; and for other races, 330.1 in 1990 and 327.4 in 1995 (Centers for Disease Control and Prevention 2006). These numbers suggest that should the dead be included in the analysis, the mean HALex of Blacks would be much lower than that of Whites and other races, and the Gini coefficient of Blacks would be much greater than that of Whites and other races. Thus, assessing health inequity between racial and ethnic groups between 1990 and 1995, we would observe less improvement for the living and dead populations combined. Based on these data, we cannot speculate whether differences in death rates between races are large enough that they offset the improvement in health equity among the living nor how they affect the overlap term of the Gini coefficient. This example reaffirms my point that health

inequity analysis should not be limited to the living but should include the dead whenever possible.

6 If one used life expectancy as the measure of health, one way to measure health inequity as health inequality by gender (as opposed to biological sex) would be to establish a norm or benchmark, for example, the smallest male-female difference in life expectancy (as a percentage of female life expectancy) observed to date. This approach can use the Shortfalls in Achievement (see sec. 4.4, Comparison, and app. A.1) as the measure of inequity.

7 I discuss in the next section more philosophical theory-oriented versions of the view of health inequity as health inequality caused by socio-economic status.

8 How best to categorize income distribution in reflecting Rawls's idea is another unsolved issue. Here I assume that my categorization is reasonable.

9 Because the decomposition technique is still in its infancy, age group stratification might further complicate the analysis. As in the case of analyses using the view of health inequity as health inequality associated with specific group characteristic, I limit the analysis in this section to all ages combined.

10 Upon defining the minimally adequate level of health, one of the fundamental questions is the relativity of the minimally adequate level of health, that is, whether there is a universal standard that applies to every person irrespective of age, sex, society, and time. The last two factors pose difficult questions especially when health inequity is analysed internationally or with a long time interval. Should we, for example, set the same minimally adequate level of health for the United States (Disability-adjusted life expectancy at birth for 1997 and 1999 is 70 years) and Sierra Leone (25.9 years) (World Health Organization 2000a)? Do we expect the same minimally adequate level of health for Americans who lived around 1900 and 2000?

11 Note that we are here referring to weights in the additively decomposable poverty measures, and we are not concerned whether one should weight-in analysis of survey data or whether inequality measures should be sensitive to the subpopulation size.

12 The Japanese analysis introduced here is reported in Asada and Ohkusa (2004).

13 See, for example, *Household Shares of Aggregate Income by Fifths of the Income Distribution: 1967 to 2001* (US Census Bureau 2002).

14 Suppose we have subpopulation $k = 1,2,...,n$. The Index of Disparity (ID)

used by Keppel, Pearcy, and Wagener (2002) is defined as follows:

$ID = \sum_{k=1}^{n} \frac{|R_k - R_t|}{n \cdot R_t} \cdot 100$, where R_k is the subgroup rate, R_t is the total

population rate, and n is the total number of subpopulations. The ID expresses the differences between the subpopulation rates as a percentage of the total population rate.

15 With the increasing understanding of poverty as a multi-dimensional concept, poverty analysis begins to focus on variables other than income. Sahn and Stifel, for example, looked at malnutrition as a poverty analysis (2002). Their study still does not give comparable results to the analysis in part 2 due to the different definition of the threshold and their focus on developing countries.

7. Conclusion

1 Daniels, Kennedy, and Kawachi argue that the answer to this question should be left to the democratic process (2000). Mooney and Jan also argue the importance of procedural justice in defining health equity (1997).

Appendices

1. See Anand et al. (2001), Anand and Sen (1994; 1995), and United Nations Development Program (2001, 240).
2. To simplify the argument, I use a slightly different version of the WHO health inequality index in this section. The WHO health inequality index used in *The World Health Report 2000* is as follows:

$W = 1 - \dfrac{\sum_{i=1}^{n} \sum_{j=1}^{n} |y_i - y_j|^{\alpha}}{2n^2 \mu^{\beta}}$. The reason why Gakidou, Murray, and Frenk

used the above is because of their desire to measure health equality instead of inequality (World Health Organization 2000a, 147). In this measure, perfect equality is one, while its variation we focus on in this section gives zero to perfect equality.
3 A debt is often expressed as negative income.
4 This is for the living population. If the population examined includes the dead, the lower anchor value of the HALex is of course zero.
5 The following explanation of the bootstrap method is adapted from Efron and Gong (1983), Efron and Tibshirani (1993), and McCarthy and

Snowden (1985). Chernick (1999) and Efron and Tibshirani (1993) provide good introductions to the bootstrap method.

6 With a sample size of more than 100,000, one can make an argument whether 95% confidence intervals are reasonable. I here, however, follow the standard practice of 95% confidence intervals without further discussing this issue.

7 See, for example, Kaufman (2000), McCarthy and Snowden (1985), Nixon et al. (1998), Rao and Wu (1988), Rust and Rao (1996), Shao and Tu (1995), Sitter (1992), and Spencer (1984).

8 For BWR, see McCarthy and Snowden (1985) and Sitter (1992). I use the INEQERR program (Jolliffe and Krushelnytskyy 1999) of Stata (StataCorp 1999b).

9 I adapt this expression from Lambert and Aronson (1993). I use the GINI-DESC program (Aliaga and Montoya 1999) of Stata (StataCorp 1999b).

10 Suppose we decompose the total Gini coefficient, G, for a population, consisting of two perfectly identical subpopulations 1 and 2. In this case, the between-group Gini coefficient is zero, and the within-group Gini coefficient for subpopulation 1 equals the within-group Gini coefficient for subpopulation 2. Recall the Population Principle: the union of populations with the same distributional pattern and the mean, that is, replication, has no effect on the degree of inequality. Because the Gini coefficient satisfies this principle, the following must be true: $G = \sum a_1 G_1 = \sum a_2 G_2$. There fore, when subpopulations are perfectly identical, despite the fact that there is (indeed, perfect) overlap, the overlap term, G_O has to be zero.

11 When $G_O = 0$, whether subpopulations perfectly overlap or do not overlap can be easily checked by looking at the between-group Gini coefficient. When subpopulations do not overlap, $G_B > 0$, while subpopulations perfectly overlap, $G_B = 0$.

12 The World Bank's *Poverty Manual* gives an excellent review of both of the FGT and SST measures (Khandker et al. 2005).

13 The SST measure is also said to be 'decomposable' (for example, Myles and Picot 2000; Xu and Osberg 2001), but one should be cautious about the way in which it is decomposable. When the SST measure's decomposition is claimed, it means that it can be decomposed into head-count ratio, gap, and inequality among people below the threshold. This is not decomposition by subpopulation group we are interested in here.

14 The Gini coefficient is decomposable but not additively decomposable, thus, its decomposition has the overlap term.

15 In this section, I follow the explanation by Foster, Greer, and Thorbecke (1984). .

16 I use the POVDECO program (Jenkins 1999) of Stata (StataCorp 1999b).

References

Acheson, Donald. 1998. *Independent inquiry into inequalities in health (The Acheson Report)*. The Stationery Office (UK). http://www.archive.official-documents.co.uk/document/doh/ih/contents.htm (accessed 27 June 2006).

Adler, Nancy E., Thomas Boyce, Margaret A. Chesney, Sheldon Cohen, Susan Folkman, Robert L. Kahn, and S. Leonard Syme. 1994. Socioeconomic status and health: The challenge of the gradient. *American Psychologist* 49:15–24.

Adler, Nancy E., Thomas Boyce, Margaret A. Chesney, Susan Folkman, and Leonard Syme. 1993. Socioeconomic inequalities in health: No easy solution. *JAMA* 269:3140–5.

Aliaga, Roger, and Silvia Montoya. 1999. GINIDESC: Stata module to compute Gini Index with within-and between-group inequality decomposition. IDEAS at the Department of Economics, College of Liberal Arts and Sciences, University of Connecticut. http://ideas.repec.org/c/boc/bocode/s372901.html (27 June 2006).

Allen, David B, and Norm Fost. 1990. Growth hormone therapy for short stature: Panacea or pandora's box? *Journal of Pediatrics* 117:16–21.

Allotey, Pascale, Daniel Reidpath, Aka Kouame, and Robert Cummins. 2003. The DALY, context and the determinants of the severity of disease: an exploratory comparison of paraplegia in Australia and Cameroon. *Social Science and Medicine* 57:949–58.

Almeida, Celia, Paula Braveman, Martha R. Gold, Célia L. Szwarcwald, José Mendres Ribeiro, Americo Miglionico, John S. Millar, Silvia Porto, Nilson do Rosário Costa, Vincente Ortun Rubio, Malcom Segall, Barbara Starfield, Cláudia Travessos, Alicia Ugá, Joaquim Valente, and Francisco Viacava. 2001. Methodological concerns and recommendations on policy consequences of the World Health Report 2000. *The Lancet* 357:1692–7.

Amiel, Y. and F.A. Cowell. 1992. Measurement of income inequality. Experimental test by questionnaire. *Journal of Public Economics* 47:3–26.

Amiel, Yoram, and Frank Cowell. 1998. Distributional orderings and the transfer principle: A re-examination. *Research on Economic Inequality* 8:195–215.

Anand, Paul. 2005. Capabilities and health. *Journal of Medical Ethics* 31:299–303.

Anand, Sudhir. 2002. The concern for equity in health. *Journal of Epidemiology and Community Health* 56:485–7.

Anand, Sudhir, Finn Diderichsen, Timothy Evans, Vladimir M. Shkolnikov, and Meg Wirth. 2001. Measuring disparities in health: Methods and indicators. In *Challenging inequalities in health: From ethics to action*, ed. T. Evans, M. Whitehead, F. Diderichsen, A. Bhuiya and M. Wirth. New York: Oxford University Press.

Anand, Sudhir, and Amartya Sen. 1994. Human Development Index: Methodology and measurement. *Human Development Report Office (HDRO), Occasional Papers* 12. <http://gd.tuwien.ac.at/soc/undp/occ.htm> (27 June 2006).

– 1995. Gender inequality in human development: Theories and measurement. *Human Development Report Office (HDRO), Occasional Papers* 19. http://gd.tuwien.ac.at/soc/undp/oc19a.htm (June 27, 2006).

Anderson, Elizabeth S. 1999. What is the point of equality? *Ethics* 109:287–337.

Anderson, Robert N. 1999. Method for constructing complete annual U.S. life tables. *Vital and Health Statistics, Series 2: Data Evaluation and Methods Research* 129. http://www.cdc.gov/nchs/data/series/sr_02/sr02_129.pdf (28 June 2006).

Anderson, Robert N., Kenneth D. Kochanek, and Sherry L. Murphy. 1997. Report of final mortality statistics, 1995. *Monthly Vital Statistics Report* 45:1–80. http://www.cdc.gov/nchs/data/mvsr/supp/mv45_11s2.pdf (27 June 2006).

Antonovsky, Aaron. 1967. Social class, life expectancy and overall mortality. *Milbank Memorial Fund Quarterly* 45:31–73.

Arneson, Richard. 1989. Equality and equal opportunity for welfare. *Philosophical Studies* 56:77–93.

– 2002. Egalitarianism. In *Stanford Encyclopedia of Philosophy* ed. E.N. Zalta. http://plato.stanford.edu/archives/fall2002/entries/egalitarianism/ (27 June 2006).

Asada, Yukiko. 2005. Assessment of the health of Americans: The average health-related quality of life and its inequality across individuals and groups. *Population Health Metrics* 3. http://www.pophealthmetrics.com/content/3/1/7 (27 June 2006).

– 2006. Is health inequality across individuals of moral concern? *Health Care Analysis* 14:25–36.

Asada, Yukiko, and Thomas Hedemann. 2002. A problem with the individual approach in the WHO health inequality measurement. *International Journal for Equity in Health* 1. http://www.equityhealthj.com/content/1/1/2 (27 June 2006).

Asada, Yukiko, and Yasushi Ohkusa. 2004. Analysis of health-related quality of life (HRQL), its distribution, and its distribution by income in Japan, 1989 and 1998. *Social Science and Medicine* 59:1423–33.

Atkinson, A.B. 1970. On the measurement on inequality. *Journal of Economic Theory* 2:244–63.

– 1983. *The economics of inequality*. 2d ed. Oxford: Clarendon Press.

Badgley, R.F. 1991. Socio and economic disparities under Canadian health care. *International Journal of Health Services* 21:659–71.

Bandourian, Ripsy. 2000. Income distributions: A comparison across countries and time. *Luxembourg Income Study Working Paper* 231. http://www.lisproject.org/publications/liswps/231.pdf (27 June 2006).

Berlin, Isaiah. 1969. Historical inevitability. In *Four essays on liberty*. Oxford: Oxford University Press.

Black, Douglas, J.N. Morris, Cyril Smith, and Peter Townsend. 1992. The Black report. In *Inequalities in health*, ed. P. Townsend and N. Davidson. London: Penguin Books.

Bleichrodt, Han, and Eddy van Doorslaer. 2006. A welfare economics foundation for health inequality measurement. *Journal of Health Economics* 25:945–57.

Bommier, Antoine, and Guy Stecklov. 2002. Defining health inequality: Why Rawls succeeds where social welfare theory fails. *Journal of Health Economics* 21:497–513.

Bossert, Walter, and Andreas Pfingsten. 1990. Intermediate inequality: Concepts, indices and welfare implications. *Mathematical Social Science* 19:117–34.

Botman, S.L., T.F. Moore, C.L. Moriarity, and V.L. Parsons. 2000. Design and estimation for the National Health Interview Survey, 1995–2004. *Vital and Health Statistics, Series 2: Data Evaluation and Methods Research* 130. http://www.cdc.gov/nchs/data/series/sr_02/sr02_130.pdf (28 June 2006).

Braveman, Paula. 2001. Epidemiology and (neo-)colonialism. *Journal of Epidemiology and Community Health* 55:160.

– 2006. Health disparities and health equity: Concepts and measurement. *Annual Review of Public Health* 27:167–94.

Braveman, Paula, and Sofia Gruskin. 2003a. Defining equity in health. *Journal of Epidemiology and Community Health* 57:254–8.

– 2003b. Poverty, equity, human rights and health. *Bulletin of the World Health Organization* 81:539–45.

Braveman, Paula, Nancy Krieger, and John Lynch. 2000. Health inequalities and social inequalities in health. *Bulletin of the World Health Organization* 78:232–3.

Braveman, Paula, Barbara Starfield, and H. Jack Geiger. 2001. World Health Report 2000: How it removes equity from the agenda for public health monitoring and policy. *BMJ* 323:678–81.

Braveman, Paula, and Eleuther Tarimo. 2002. Social inequalities in health within countries: Not only an issue for affluent nations. *Social Science and Medicine* 54:1621–35.

Brock, Dan W. 2000. Broadening the bioethics agenda. *Kennedy Institute of Ethics Journal* 10:21–38.

Broome, John. 1989. What's the good of equality? In *Current issues in microeconomics*, ed. J. Hey. London: Palgrave Macmillan.

– Forthcoming. Equality versus priority: A useful distinction. In *Health, well being, justice: Ethical issues in health resource allocation*, ed. D. Wikler and C. Murray. In preparation.

Brouwer, Werner B.F., Job A. van Exel, and Elly A. Stolk. 2005. Acceptability of less than perfect health states. *Social Science and Medicine* 60:237–46.

Buchanan, Allen E. 1984. The right to a decent minimum of health care. *Philosophy and Public Affairs* 13:55–78.

Bureau of Labor Statistics, and Bureau of the Census. 2001. *Current Population Survey* 4 April 2001. http://www.bls.census.gov/cps/cpsmain.htm (28 June 2006).

Callahan, Daniel. 1987. *Setting limits.* New York: Simon & Schuster.

Cappelen, Alexander W., and Ole Frithjof Norheim. 2005. Responsibility in health care: A liberal egalitarian approach. *Journal of Medical Ethics* 31:476–80.

– 2006. Responsibility, fairness and rationing in health care. *Health Policy* 76:312–19.

Carr-Hill, Roy, and Paul Chalmers-Dixon. 2005. The public health observatory handbook of health inequalities measurement. Oxford, UK: South East Public Health Observatory. http://www.sepho.org.uk/extras/rch_handbook.aspx (27 June 2006).

Cater-Pokras, Olivia, and Claudia Baquet. 2002. What is a 'health disparity'? *Public Health Reports* 117:426–34.

Centers for Disease Control and Prevention. 2006. *CDC Wonder*, 14 March 2006. http://wonder.cdc.gov/ (27 June 2006).

Chang, W.C. 2002. The meaning and goals of equity in health. *Journal of Epidemiology and Community Health* 56:488–91.

Charlton, Bruce G. 1994. Is inequality bad for the national health? *The Lancet* 343:221–2.

Chatterji, Somnath, Bedirhan L. Üstün, Joshua A. Salomon, Colin D. Mathers, and Christopher J. L. Murray. 2002. The conceptual basis for measuring and reporting on health. *Global Programme on Evidence for Health Policy Discussion Paper* 45. http://www3.who.int/whosis/discussion_papers/discussion_papers.cfm?path=whosis,evidence, discussion_papers&language=english (27 June 2006).

Chernick, Michael R. 1999. *Bootstrap methods: A practitioner's guide, Wiley Series in Probability and Statistics.* New York: Wiley-Interscience Publication.

Clarke, Philip M., Ulf-G. Gerdtham, and Luke B. Connelly. 2003. A note on the decomposition of the health concentration index. *Health Economics* 12: 511–16.

Clarke, Philip M., Ulf-G. Gerdtham, Magnus Johannesson, Kerstin Bingefors, and Len Smith. 2002. On the measurement of relative and absolute income-related health inequality. *Social Science and Medicine* 55:1923–8.

Coulter, Philip B. 1989. *Measuring inequality: A methodological handbook.* Boulder, CO: Westview Press.

Cowell, F.A. 1995. *Measuring inequality.* 2nd ed. London: Prentice Hall/Harvester Wheatsheaf.

– 2000. Measurement of inequality. In *Handbook of income distribution,* ed. A.B. Atkinson and F. Burguignon. Amsterdam: Elsevier.

Culyer, A.J., and Adam Wagstaff. 1993. Equity and equality in health and health care. *Journal of Health Economics* 12:431–57.

Culyer, Anthony J. 2001. Equity – some theory and its policy implications. *Journal of Medical Ethics* 27:275–83.

Cutler, David M., and Elizabeth Richardson. 1997. Measuring the health of the U.S. population. *Brookings Papers on Economic Activity. Microeconomics* 1997:217–71.

Dagum, C. 1997. A new approach to the decomposition of the Gini income inequality ratio. *Empirical Economics* 22:515–31.

Dalton, Hugh. 1920. The measurement of the inequality of incomes. *Economic Journal* 30:348–61.

Daniels, Norman. 1985. *Just health care.* Cambridge: Cambridge University Press.

– 1988. *Am I my parents' keeper?* Oxford: Oxford University Press.

Daniels, Norman, Bruce Kennedy, and Ichiro Kawachi. 2000. *Is inequality bad for our health?* Boston: Beacon Press.

– 2004. Health and inequality, or, why justice is good for our health. In *Public health, ethics, and equity,* ed. S. Anand, F. Peter and A. Sen. Oxford: Oxford University Press.

Deaton, Angus. 1997. *The analysis of household surveys: A microeconometric approach to development policy.* Baltimore and London: Published for the World Bank, the Johns Hopkins University Press.

— 2002. Policy implications of the gradient of health and wealth. *Health Affairs* 21:13–30.

Dolan, Paul, and Jan Able Olsen. 2001. Equity in health: The importance of different health streams. *Journal of Health Economics* 20:823–34.

Dolan, Paul, and Rebecca Shaw. 2001. How much do people care about health inequalities? *Health Variations: The Official Newsletter of the ESRC Health Variations Programme* 7:14–15. http://www.lancs.ac.uk/fss/apsocsci/hvp/newsletters/dolan7.htm (27 June 2006).

Drummond, Michael F., Bernie O'Brien, Greg L. Stoddart, and George W. Torrance. 1997. *Methods for the economic evaluation of health care programmes.* 2d ed. Oxford: Oxford University Press.

Dutta, B. and J.M. Esteban. 1991. Social welfare and equality. *Social Choice and Welfare* 9:267–76.

Dworkin, Ronald. 1981a. What is equality? Part 1: Equality of welfare. *Philosophy and Public Affairs* 10:185–246.

— 1981b. What is equality? Part 2: Equality of resources. *Philosophy and Public Affairs* 10:283–345.

Efron, B., and G. Gong. 1983. A leisurely look at the bootstrap, the jackknife and cross-validation. *American Statistician* 37:36–48.

Efron, Bradley, and Robert J. Tibshirani. 1993. *An introduction to the bootstrap.* Boca Raton, FL: Chapman & Hall/CRC.

Erickson, P. 1998. Evaluation of a population-based measure of quality of life – The Health and Activity Limitation Index (Halex). *Quality of Life Research* 7:101–14.

Erickson, Pennifer, Ronald Wilson, and Ildy Shannon. 1995. Years of Health Life. *Healthy People 2000, Statistical Notes* 7. http://www.cdc.gov/nchs/data/statnt/statnt07.pdf (27 June 2006).

Evans, Robert G., Morris L. Barer, and Theodore R. Marmor, eds. 1994. *Why are some people healthy and others not? The determinants of health of populations.* New York: Aldine De Gruyter.

Evans, Robert G., and Gregory L. Stoddart. 1990. Producing health, consuming health care. *Social Science and Medicine* 31:1347–63.

Families USA. 2003. Going without health insurance: Nearly one in three non-elderly Americans. Washington, DC: Families USA. http://www.familiesusa.org/assets/pdfs/Going_without_report3b26.pdf (27 June 2006).

Feeny, David, William Furlong, Michael Boyle, and George W. Torrance. 1995. Multi-attribute health status classification systems: Health Utilities Index. *PharmacoEconomics* 7:490–502.

Feeny, David, William Furlong, George W. Torrance, Charles H. Goldsmith, Zenlong Zhu, Sonja DePauw, Margaret Denton, and Michael Boyle. 2002. Multi-attribute and single-attribute utility functions for the Health Utilities Index Mark 3 system. *Medical Care* 40:113–28.

Feinstein, Jonathan S. 1993. The relationship between socioeconomic status and health: A review of the literature. *Milbank Quarterly* 71:279–322.

Feminist Health Care Ethics Research Network, Susan Sherwin, Francoise Baylis, Marilynne Bell, Maria De Koninck, Jocelyn Downie, Abby Lippman, Margaret Lock, Wendy Mitchinson, Mathryn Pauly Morgan, Janet Mosher, and Barbara Parish. 1998. *The politics of women's health.* Philadelphia: Temple University Press.

Ferrer, R.L., and R. Palmer. 2004. Variations in health status within and between socioeconomic strata. *Journal of Epidemiology and Community Health* 58:381–7.

Field, Marilyn J., and Marthe R. Gold, eds. 1998. Committee on Summary Measures of Population Health, Institute of Medicine. *Summarizing population health: Directions for the development and application of population metrics.* Washington, DC: National Academy Press. http://darwin.nap.edu/books/0309060990/html/1.html (27 June 2006).

Fleurbaey, Marc. Forthcoming (a). Equality versus priority: How relevant is the distinction? In *Health, well being, justice: Ethical issues in health resource allocation,* ed. D. Wikler and C. Murray. In preparation.

Fleurbaey, Marc. Forthcoming (b). On the measurement of health and of health inequalities. In *Health, well being, justice: Ethical issues in health resource allocation,* ed. D. Wikler and C. Murray. In preparation.

Foster, J., J. Greer, and E. Thorbecke. 1984. A class of decomposable poverty measures. *Econometrica* 52:761–5.

Foster, James E. 1985. Inequality measurement. *American Mathematical Society* 33:31–69.

Foster, James E., and Artyom A. Shneyerov. 2000. Path independent inequality measures. *Journal of Economic Theory* 91:199–222.

Freeman, Harold P., and Richard Payne. 2000. Racial injustice in health care. *New England Journal of Medicine* 342:1045–7.

Froberg, Debra G., and Robert L. Kane. 1989a. Methodology for measuring health-state preferences – I: Measurement strategies. *Journal of Clinical Epidemiology* 42:345–54.

– 1989b. Methodology for measuring health-state preferences – II: Scaling methods. *Journal of Clinical Epidemiology* 42:459–71.

– 1989c. Methodology for measuring health-state preferences – III: Population and context effects. *Journal of Clinical Epidemiology* 42:585–92.

– 1989d. Methodology for measuring health-state preferences – IV: Progress and a research agenda. *Journal of Clinical Epidemiology* 42:675–85.

Fryback, Dennis G. 1998. Appendix C: Methodological issues in measuring health status and health-related quality of life for population health measures: A brief overview of the 'HALY' family of measures. In *Summarizing population health: Directions for the development and application of population metrics*, ed. M.J. Field and M.R. Gold. Washington, DC: National Academy Press.

Frye, Marilyn. 1983. Oppression. In *The Politics of Reality*. Freedom: The Crossing Press.

Gakidou, Emmanuela E., and Gary King. 2002. Measuring total health inequality: Adding individual variation to group-level differences. *International Journal for Equity in Health* 1. http://www.equityhealthj.com/content/pdf/1475–9276–1–3.pdf (27 June 2006).

Gakidou, Emmanuela E., Christopher J.L. Murray, and Julio Frenk. 2000. Defining and measuring health inequality: An approach based on the distribution of health expectancy. *Bulletin of the World Health Organization* 78:42–54.

– 2001. Measuring preferences on health system performance assessment. *Global Programme on Evidence for Health Policy Discussion Paper* 20. http://www3.who.int/whosis/discussion_papers/discussion_papers.cfm?path=whosis,evidence, discussion_papers&language=english (27 June 2006).

Galea, Sandro, Jennifer Ahern, and Adam Karpati. 2005. A model of underlying socioeconomic vulnerability in human populations: Evidence from variability in population health and implications for public health. *Social Science and Medicine* 60:2417–30.

Gold, Marthe R., David Stevenson, and Dennis G. Fryback. 2002. HALYs and QALYs and DALYs, oh my: Similarities and differences in summary measure of population health. *Annual Review of Public Health* 23:115–34.

Goldman, Noreen. 2001. Social inequalities in health: Disentangling the underlying mechanisms. *Annals of the New York Academy of Sciences* 954:118–39.

Gordis, Leon. 1996. *Epidemiology*. Philadelphia: W.B. Saunders.

Gosepath, Stefan. 2001. Equality. In *Stanford Encyclopedia of Philosophy*, ed. E.N. Zalta. http://plato.stanford.edu/archives/win2001/entries/equality/ (27 June 2006).

Graham, Hilary. 2004. Social determinants and their unequal distribution: Clarifying policy understandings. *Milbank Quarterly* 82:101–24.

Greenacre, Michael. 1992. Correspondence analysis in medical research. *Statistical Methods in Medical Research* 1:97–117.

– 2002. Correspondence analysis of the Spanish National Health Survey. *Gaceta Sanitaria* 16:160–70.

Griffin, James. Forthcoming. A human right to health. In *Health, well being, justice: Ethical issues in health resource allocation*, ed. D. Wikler and C. Murray. In preparation.

Gunning-Schepers, Louise J., and Karien Stronks. 1999. Inequalities in health: Future threats to equity. *Acta Oncologica* 38:57–61.

Gwatkin, Davidson R. 2000. Health in equalities and the health of the poor: What do we know? What can we do? *Bulletin of the World Health Organization* 78:3–18.

Gwatkin, Davidson R., Michel Guillot, and Patrick Heuveline. 1999. The burden of disease among the global poor. *The Lancet* 354:586–9.

Gwatkin, Davidson R., and Patrick Heuveline. 1999. Improving the health of the world's poor. *BMJ* 315:497–8.

Hall, Wayne. 1986. Social class and survival on the S.S. *Titanic*. *Social Science and Medicine* 22:687–90.

Harper, Sam, and John Lynch. 2005. *Methods for measuring cancer disparities: Using data relevant to* Healthy People 2010 *cancer-related objectives*. National Cancer Institute Cancer Surveillance Monograph Series, no. 6. Bethesda, MD: National Cancer Institute. http://seer.cancer.gov/publications/disparities/measuring_disparities.pdf (27 June 2006).

Harris, John. 1999. Justice and equal opportunities in health care. *Bioethics* 13:392–404.

Harrison, E., and C. Seidl. 1994. Perceptional inequality and preferential judgments: An empirical examination of distributional axioms. *Public Choice* 79:61–81.

Hausman, Daniel M. 2002. The limits to empirical ethics. In *Summary measures of population health: Concepts, ethics, measurement and applications*, ed. C.J.L. Murray, J.A. Salomon, C.D. Mathers, and A.D. Lopez. Geneva: World Health Organization.

– 2006. Valuing health. *Philosophy and Public Affairs* 34:246–74.

– 2007. What's wrong with health inequalities? *Journal of Political Philosophy* 15: 46–66.

– Forthcoming – a. Equality versus priority: A badly misleading distinction. In *Health, well being, justice: Ethical issues in health resource allocation*, ed. D. Wikler and C. Murray. In preparation.

Hausman, Daniel M., Yukiko Asada, and Thomas Hedemann. 2002. Health inequalities and why they matter. *Health Care Analysis* 10:177–91.

Hausman, Daniel M., and Michael S. McPherson. 2006. *Economic analysis, moral philosophy and public policy*. 2d ed. New York: Cambridge University Press.

Health Canada. 1996. Towards a common understanding: Clarifying the core concepts of population health. *Discussion paper* H39–391/1996E. http://

www.phac-aspc.gc.ca/ph-sp/phdd/docs/common/index.html (27 June 2006).

Health Inequalities in Modern Societies and Beyond. 1997. *Social Science and Medicine* 44 (6).

Heinrich, Georges A. 1998. The prince and the pauper revisited: A bootstrap approach to poverty and income distribution analysis using the PACO data base. *International Networks for Studies in Technology, Environment, Alternatives, Development PACO research paper* 21.

Hertzman, Clyde, John Frank, and Robert G. Evans. 1994. Heterogeneities in health status and the determinants of population health. In *Why Are Some People Healthy And Others Not?* ed. R.G. Evans, M.L. Barer and T.R. Marmor. New York: Aldine De Gruyter.

Hosseinpoor, Ahmad Reza, Kazem Mohammad, Reza Majdzadeh, Mohsen Naghavi, Farid Abolhassani, Angelica Sousa, Niko Speybroeck, Hamid Reza Jamshidi, and Jeanette Vega. 2005. Socioeconomic inequality in infant mortality in Iran and across its provinces. *Bulletin of the World Health Organization* 83:837–44.

House, James S., Ronald C. Kessler, A. Regula Herzog, Richard P. Mero, Ann M. Kinney, and Martha J. Breslow. 1990. Age, socioeconomic status, and health. *Milbank Quarterly* 68:383–411.

Howes, Stephen, and Jean Olson Lanjouw. 1998. Does sample design matter for poverty rate comparisons? *Review of Income and Wealth* 44:99–109.

Humphries, Karin H., and Eddy van Doorslaer. 2000. Income-related health inequality in Canada. *Social Science and Medicine* 50:663–71.

Idler, E.L., and S.V. Kasl. 1995. Self-ratings of health: Do they also predict change in functional ability? *Journal of Gerontology* 50:S344–53.

Illsley, Raymond, and Julian Le Grand. 1987. Measurement of inequality in health. In *Health in economics*, ed. A. Williams. London: Macmillan.

Inequalities in health. 2000. *Bulletin of the World Health Organization* 78(1).

Jefferson, Thomas. 1787. To T.M. Randolph, Jr. (Paris). In *The Jeffersonian cyclopedia: A comprehensive collection of the views of Thomas Jefferson (1900)*, ed. J.P. Foley. New York and London: Funk & Wagnalls Company. http://etext.lib. virginia.edu/jefferson/quotations/foley/ (27 June 2006).

Jenkins, Stephen P. 1999. POVDECO: Stata module to calculate poverty indices with decomposition by subgroup. IDEAS at the Department of Economics, College of Liberal Arts and Sciences, University of Connecticut. http://ideas.repec.org/c/boc/bocode/s366004.html (29 December 2006).

Jolliffe, Dean, and Bohdan Krushelnytskyy. 1999. Bootstrap standard errors for indices of inequality: INEQERR. *Stata Technical Bulletin* 51.

Jolliffe, Dean, and Anastassia Semykina. 1999. Robust standard errors for the Foster-Greer-Thorbecke class of poverty indices: SEPOV. *Stata Technical Bulletin* 51.

Kakwani, Nanak C. 1980. *Income inequality and poverty: Methods of estimation and policy applications.* Oxford: Oxford University Press (published for the World Bank).

Kakwani, Nanak C., Adam Wagstaff, and Eddy van Doorslaer. 1997. Socioeconomic inequalities in health: Measurement, computation, and statistical inference. *Journal of Econometrics* 77:87–103.

Kaplow, Louis. 2002. Why measure inequality? *National Bureau of Economic Research Working Paper* 9342. http://www.nber.org/papers/w9342 (27 June 2006).

Karagiannis, Elias, and Milorad Kovacevic. 2000. A method to calculate the jackknife variance estimator for the Gini coefficient. *Oxford Bulletin of Economics and Statistics* 62:119–22.

Kaufman, Steven. 2000. Using the bootstrap to estimate the variance in a very complex sample design. Paper read at Proceedings of the Survey Research Methods Section, American Statistical Association.

Kawachi, I., S.V. Subramanian, and N. Almeida-Filho. 2002. A glossary for health inequalities. *Journal of Epidemiology and Community Health* 56:647–52.

Kawachi, Ichiro, Norman Daniels, and Dean Robinson. 2005. Health disparities by race and class: Why both matter. *Health Affairs* 24:343–52.

Kawachi, Ichiro, Bruce P. Kennedy, and Richard G. Wilkinson, eds. 1999. *Income inequality and health.* Vol. 1. The Society and Population Health Reader. New York: New Press.

Kekes, John. 1997. A question for egalitarians. *Ethics* 107:658–69.

Keppel, Kenneth G., Elsie Pamuk, John Lynch, Olivia Carter-Pokras, Insun Kim, Vickie Mays, Jeffrey Pearcy, Victor Schoenbach, and Joel S. Weissman. 2005. Methodological issues in measuring health disparities. *Vital and Health Statistics* 2. http://www.cdc.gov/nchs/data/series/sr_02/sr02_141.pdf (27 June 2006).

Keppel, Kenneth G., Jeffrey N. Pearcy, and Richard J. Klein. 2004. Measuring progress in *Healthy People 2010. Healthy People 2000, Statistical Notes* 25. http://www.cdc.gov/nchs/data/statnt/statnt25.pdf (27 June 2006).

Keppel, Kenneth G., Jeffrey N. Pearcy, and Diane K. Wagener. 2002. Trends in racial and ethnic-specific rates for the health status indicators: United States, 1990–98. *Healthy People 2000: Statistical Notes* 23. http://www.cdc.gov/nchs/data/statnt/statnt23.pdf (27 June 2006).

Khandker, Shahid, Jonathan Haughton, Kathleen Beegle, Celia Reyes, and Nidhiya Menon. 2005. Poverty manual: Introduction to poverty analysis.

Washington, DC: World Bank. http://siteresources.worldbank.org/PGLP/
Resources/PovertyManual.pdf (28 June 2006).

Kolm, Serge-Christophe. 1976. Unequal inequalities II. *Journal of Economic Theory* 13:82–111.

– Forthcoming. On health and justice. In *Health, well being, justice: Ethical issues in health resource allocation*, ed D. Wikler and C.J.L. Murray. In preparation.

Koolman, Xander, and Eddy van Doorslaer. 2004. On the interpretation of a concentration index of inequality. *Health Economics* 13:649–56.

Lahelma, Eero, Katariina Kivela, Eva Roos, Terhi Tuominen, Espen Dahl, Finn Diderichsen, Jon Ivar Elstad, Inge Lissau, Olle Lundberg, Ossi Rahkonen, Niels Kristian Rasmussen, and Monica Aberg Yngwe. 2002. Analyzing changes of health inequalities in the Nordic welfare states. *Social Science and Medicine* 55:609–25.

Lalonde, Marc. 1974. A new perspective on the health of Canadians: A working document. Ottawa: Government of Canada. http://www.hc-sc.gc.ca/hcs-sss/com/lalonde/index_e.html (28 June 2006).

Lambert, Peter J., and J. Richard Aronson. 1993. Inequality decomposition analysis and the Gini coefficient revisited. *Economic Journal* 103:1221–7.

Le Grand, J. 1987. Inequality in health: Some international comparison. *European Economic Review* 31:182–91.

Le Grand, Julian. 1991. *Equity and choice: An essay in economics and applied philosophy*. London: HarperCollins Academic.

Leon, David A., Gill Walt, and Lucy Gilson. 2001. International perspectives on health inequalities and policy. *BMJ* 322:591–4.

Levins, Richard, and Cynthia Lopez. 1999. Toward an ecosocial view of health. *International Journal of Health Services* 29:261–93.

Levy, Jonathan I., Susan M. Chemerynski, and Jessica L. Tuchmann. 2006. Incorporating concepts of inequality and inequity into health benefit analysis. *International Journal for Equity in Health* 5. http://www.equityhealthj.com/content/pdf/1475-9276-5-2.pdf (28 June 2006).

Lindholm, L., and M. Rosen. 1998. On the measurement of the nation's equity adjusted health. *Health Economics* 7:621–8.

Link, Bruce G., and Jo Phelan. 1995. Social conditions as fundamental causes of disease. *Journal of Health and Social Behavior* Extra issue:80–94.

Litchfield, Julie A. 1999. Inequality: methods and tools. World Bank, Inequality, Poverty, and Socio-economic Performance. http://www1.worldbank.org/prem/poverty/inequal/methods/ (28 June 2006).

Low, Allan, and Anne Low. 2006. Importance of relative measures in policy on health inequalities. *BMJ* 332:967–9.

Luxembourg Income Study. 2006. *Luxembourg Income Study key figures: Income inequality measures*, 8 June 2006. http://www.lisproject.org/keyfigures/ineqtable.htm (28 June 2006).

Lynch, John, and Sam Harper. 2005. *Measuring health disparities (CD-ROM)*. Ann Arbor: Michigan Public Health Training Center.

Lynch, John, George Davey Smith, Sam Harper, and Kathleen Bainbridge. 2006. Explaining the social gradient in coronary heart disease: Comparing relative and absolute risk approaches. *Journal of Epidemiology and Community Health* 60:436–41.

Lynch, John, George Davey Smith, Sam Harper, and Marianne Hillemeier. 2004a. Is income inequality a determinant of population health? Part 2. U.S. national and regional trends in income inequality and age-and cause-specific mortality. *Milbank Quarterly* 82:355–400.

Lynch, John, George Davey Smith, Sam Harper, Marianne Hillemeier, Nancy Ross, George A. Kaplan, and Michael Wolfson. 2004b. Is income inequality a determinant of population health? Part 1. A systematic review. *Milbank Quarterly* 82:5–99.

Machinko, James A., and Barbara Starfield. 2002. Annotated bibliography on equity in health, 1980–2001. *International Journal for Equity in Health* 1. http://www.equityhealthj.com/content/1/1/1 (28 June 2006).

Mackenbach, Johan P. 1993. Inequalities in health in the Netherlands according to age, gender, marital status, level of education, degree of urbanization, and region. *European Journal of Public Health* 3:112–18.

Mackenbach, Johan P., and Anton E. Kunst. 1997. Measuring the magnitude of socio-economic inequalities in health: An overview of available measures illustrated with two examples from Europe. *Social Science and Medicine* 44:757–71.

Mann, Jonathan M. 1997. Medicine and public health, ethics and human rights. *Hastings Center Report* 27:6–13.

Manor, Orly, Sharon Matthews, and Chris Power. 1997. Comparing measures of health inequality. *Social Science and Medicine* 45:761–71.

Marchand, Sarah, Daniel Wikler, and Bruce Landesman. 1998. Class, health, and justice. *Milbank Quarterly* 76:449–67.

Marmot, Michael. 2001. From Black to Acheson: Two decades of concern with inequalities in health. A celebration of the 90th birthday of Professor Jerry Morris. *International Journal of Epidemiology* 30:1165–71.

Massey, James T., T.F. Moore, V.L. Parsons, and W. Tadros. 1989. Design and estimation for the National Health Interview Survey, 1985–94. *Vital and Health Statistics, Series 2: Data Evaluation and Methods Research* 110.

http://www.cdc.gov/nchs/data/series/sr_02/sr02_110.pdf (28 June 2006).

Mayberry, Robert M., Fatima Mili, and Elizabeth Ofili. 2000. Racial and ethnic differences in access to medical care. *Medical Care Research and Review* 57:108–45.

McCarthy, Philip J., and Cecelia B. Snowden. 1985. The bootstrap and finite population sampling. *Vital and Health Statistics* 2. Public Health Service Publication 85–1369.

McDowell, Ian, and Claire Newll. 1996. *Measuring health: A guide to rating scales and questionnaires.* 2d ed. New York: Oxford University Press.

McIntyre, Di, and Lucy Gilson. 2002. Putting equity in health back onto the social policy agenda: Experience from South Africa. *Social Science and Medicine* 54:1637–56.

McKee, Martin. 2001. Measuring the efficiency of health systems. *BMJ* 323:295–6.

McKerlie, Dennis. 1989. Equality and time. *Ethics* 99:475–91.

– 1992. Equality between age-groups. *Philosophy and Public Affairs* 21:275–95.

– 1997. Priority and time. *Canadian Journal of Philosophy* 27:287–309.

– 2002. Justice between the young and the old. *Philosophy and Public Affairs* 30:152–77.

Mills, Jeffrey A., and Sourushe Zandvakili. 1997. Statistical inference via bootstrapping for measures of inequality. *Journal of Applied Econometrics* 12:133–50.

Mooney, Gavin, and Stephen Jan. 1997. Vertical equity: Weighting outcomes? or Establishing procedures? *Health Policy* 39:79–87.

Muntaner, Carles. 2002. Power, politics, and social class. *Journal of Epidemiology and Community Health* 56:562.

Murray, Christopher J.L. 1996. Rethinking DALYs. In *Global Burden of Disease,* ed. C.J.L. Murray and A.D. Lopez. Cambridge, MA: Harvard University Press on behalf of World Health Organization and World Bank.

Murray, Christopher J.L., Emmanuela E. Gakidou, and Julio Frenk. 1999. Health inequalities and social group differences: What should we measure? *Bulletin of the World Health Organization* 77:537–43.

– 2000. Response to P. Braveman et al. *Bulletin of the World Health Organization* 78:234.

Murray, Christopher J.L., Joshua A. Salmon, Colin D. Mathers, and Alan D. Lopez, eds. 2002. *Summary measures of population health: Concepts, ethics, measurement and applications.* Geneva: World Health Organization.

Musgrove, Philip. 1986. Measurement of equity in health. *World Health Statistics Quarterly* 39:325–35.

Mustard, C.A., and J. Etches. 2003. Gender differences in socioeconomic inequality in mortality. *Journal of Epidemiology and Community Health* 57:974–80.

Myles, John, and Garnett Picot. 2000. Poverty indices and policy analysis. *Review of Income and Wealth* 46:161–79.

National Center for Health Statistics. 1994. Vital statistics of the United States, 1990. Vol. 2, sec. 6, life tables. Washington, DC: Public Health Service. http://www.cdc.gov/nchs/data/lifetables/life90_2acc.pdf (28 June 2006).

– 1997. US decennial life tables for 1989–91. Vol. 1, no. 1, United States Life Tables. Hyattsville, MD: Public Health Service. http://www.cdc.gov/nchs/data/lifetables/life89_1_1.pdf (28 June 2006).

– 1998. Vital statistics of the United States, 1995, preprint of vol 2, mortality, part A, sec. 6, life tables. Hyattsville, MD: Public Health Service. http://www.cdc.gov/nchs/data/lifetables/life95_2.pdf (28 June 2006).

– 2001. Healthy People 2000 final review. Hyattsville, MD: Public Health Service. http://www.cdc.gov/nchs/data/hp2000/hp2k01.pdf (28 June 2006).

Navarro, Vicente. 2002. The World Health Report 2000: Can health care systems be compared using a single measure of performance? *American Journal of Public Health* 92:30–4.

Nixon, Mary Gessley, J. Michael Brick, Graham Kalton, and Hyunshik Lee. 1998. Alternative variance estimation methods for the NHIS. Paper read at Proceedings of the Survey Research Methods Section, American Statistical Association.

Norheim, Ole Frithjof. 2006. Measuring pure health inequity before and after interventions: A supplement to cost-effectiveness analysis? Unpublished manuscript. University of Bergen, Norway.

Nussbaum, Martha C. 2000. *Women and human development: The capabilities approach.* Cambridge: Cambridge University Press.

O'Neill, Onora. 2003. Trust with accountability. *Journal of Health Services Research and Policy* 8:3–4.

Ogwang, Tomson. 2000. A convenient method of computing the Gini index and its standard error. *Oxford Bulletin of Economics and Statistics* 62:123–9.

Okun, M.A., W.A. Stock, M.J. Haring, and R.A. Witter. 1984. Health and subjective well-being: A meta-analysis. *International Journal of Ageing and Human Development* 192:111–32.

Olsen, Jan Abel. 1997. Theories of justice and their implications for priority setting in health care. *Journal of Health Economics* 16:625–39.

Oppenheim, Felix. 1970. Egalitarianism as a descriptive concept. *American Philosophical Quarterly* 7:143–52.

Osberg, Lars, and Kuan Xu. 1999. Poverty intensity: How well do Canadian provinces compare? *Canadian Public Policy / Analyse de politiques* XXV: 179–95.

– 2000. International comparison of poverty intensity: Index decomposition and bootstrap Inference. *Journal of Human Resources* 35:51–81.

Pamuk, E.R. 1985. Social class and inequality in mortality in England and Wales from 1921 to 1980. *Population Studies* 39:17–31.

– 1988. Social-class inequality in infant mortality in England and Wales from 1921–1980. *European Journal of Population* 4:1–21.

Pappas, Gregory, Susan Queen, Wilbur Hadden, and Gail Fisher. 1993. The increasing disparity in mortality between socioeconomic groups in the United States, 1960 and 1986. *New England Journal of Medicine* 329:103–9.

Parfit, Derek. 1991. Equality or priority? Paper read at the Lindley Lecture, the University of Kansas, Lawrence, KS.

Pearcy, Jeffrey N., and Kenneth G. Keppel. 2002. A summary measure of health disparity. *Public Health Reports* 117:273–80.

Pereira, Joao. 1993. What does equity in health mean? *Journal of Social Policy* 22:19–48.

Peter, Fabienne. 2001. Health equity and social justice. *Journal of Applied Philosophy* 18:159–70.

Peter, Fabienne, and Timothy Evans. 2001. Ethical dimensions of health equity. In *Challenging inequalities in health: From ethics to action*, ed. T. Evans, M. Whitehead, F. Diderichsen, A. Bhuiya, and M. Wirth. New York: Oxford University Press.

Pickett, Joseph P., et al., eds. 2000. *The American heritage dictionary of the English language*. 4th ed. Boston: Houghton Mifflin.

Power, Chris, Sharon Matthews, and Orly Manor. 1998. Inequalities in self-rated health: Explanations from different stages of life. *The Lancet* 351:1009–14.

Powers, Madison, and Ruth Faden. 2000. Inequalities in health, inequalities in health care: Four generations of discussion about justice and cost-effectiveness analysis. *Kennedy Institute of Ethics Journal* 10:109–27.

Pradhan, Menno, David E. Sahn, and Stephen D. Younger. 2003. Decomposing world health inequality. *Journal of Health Economics* 22:271–93.

Public Health Agency of Canada. 2002. *What is population health?* 29 November 2002, http://www.phac-aspc.gc.ca/ph-sp/phdd/approach/index. html#What (27 June 2006).

Pyatt, Graham. 1976. On the interpretation and disaggregation of Gini coefficients. *Economic Journal* 86:243–55.

Rao, J.N.K., and C.F.J. Wu. 1988. Resampling inference with complex survey data. *Journal of the American Statistical Association* 83:231–41.

Raphael, Dennis. 2000. Health inequalities in the United States: Prospects and solutions. *Journal of Public Health Policy* 21:394–427.

Rawls, John. 1971. *A theory of justice.* Cambridge, MA: Belknap Press.

Regidor, Enrique. 2004a. Measures of health inequalities, Part 1. *Journal of Epidemiology and Community Health* 58:858–61.

– 2004b. Measures of health inequalities, Part 2. *Journal of Epidemiology and Community Health* 58:900–03.

Reidpath, Daniel D., Pascale A. Allotey, Aka Kouame, and Robert A. Cummins. 2003. Measuring health in a vacuum: Examining the disability weight of the DALY. *Health, Policy and Planning* 18:351–6.

Rio, Coral del, and Javier Ruiz-Castillo. 2000. Intermediate inequality and welfare. *Social Choice and Welfare* 17:223–39.

Robert, Stephanie A., and James S. House. 2000. Socioeconomic inequalities in health: An enduring sociological problem. In *Handbook of Medical Sociology*, ed. C.E. Bird, P. Conrad, and A.M. Fremont. Upper Saddle River, NJ: Prentice Hall.

Roemer, John E., Thomas J. Scanlon, Robert M. Solow, Samuel Scheffler, Richard A. Epstein, Elizabeth Fox-Genovese, Eric Maskin, Arthur Ripstein, S.L. Hurley, and Nancy L. Rosenblum. 1995. Social equality and personal responsibility (A debate on John Roemer's 'Equality and responsibility'). *Boston Review* 20(2) http://bostonreview.net/BR20.2/BR20.2.html.

Rose, Geoffrey. 1992. *The strategy of preventive medicine.* Oxford: Oxford University Press.

Ross, Nancy A. 2004. What have we learned studying income inequality and population health? Ottawa: Canadian Institute for Health Information. http://secure.cihi.ca/cihiweb/dispPage.jsp?cw_page=reports_e#W (28 June 2006).

Ross, Nancy A., Stéphane Tremblay, and Katie Graham. 2004. Neighbourhood influences on health in Montréal, Canada. *Social Science and Medicine* 59:1485–94.

Rust, K.F., and J.N.K. Rao. 1996. Variance estimation for complex surveys using replication techniques. *Statistical Methods in Medical Research* 5:283–310.

Sahn, David E., and David C. Stifel. 2002. Robust comparisons of malnutrition in developing countries. *American Journal of Agricultural Economics* 84:716–35.

Salomon, Joshua A., Ajay Tandon, Christopher J.L. Murray, and World Health Survey Pilot Study Collaborating Group. 2004. Comparability of self-rated health: cross sectional multi-country survey using anchoring vignettes. *BMJ* 328:258.

Salomon, Joshua A., Colin D. Mathers, Somnath Chatterji, Ritu Sadana, T. Bedirhan Üstün, and Christopher J.L. Murray. 2003. Quantifying individual levels of health: Definitions, concepts, and measurement issues. In *Health Systems Performance Assessment: Debates, Methods and Empiricism*, ed. C.J.L. Murray and D.B. Evans. Geneva: World Health Organization.

Seidl, Christian, and Andreas Pfingsten. 1997. Ray invariant inequality measures. In *Inequality and Taxation*, ed. S. Zandvakili. Greenwich, CT, and London: JAI Press.

Sen, Amartya. 1976. Poverty: An ordinal approach to measurement. *Econometrica* 44:219–31.

– 1992. *Inequality reexamined*. Cambridge, MA: Harvard University Press.

– 1993. Capability and well-being. In *The quality of life*, ed. M. Nussbaum and A. Sen. Oxford: Clarendon Press.

– 1997. *On economic inequality*. Expanded edition with a substantial annex by James E. Foster and Amartya Sen. Oxford: Oxford University Press.

– 1998. Mortality as an indicator of economic success and failure. *Economic Journal* 108:1–25.

– 2002a. Health: Perception versus observation. *BMJ* 324:860–1.

– 2002b. Why health equity? *Health Economics* 11:659–66.

Shao, Jun, and Dongsheng Tu. 1995. Chapter 6: Applications to sample surveys. In *The Jackknife and Bootstrap*. New York: Springer.

Shibuya, Kenji, Hideki Hashimoto, and Eiji Yano. 2002. Individual income, income distribution, and self rated health in Japan: Cross-sectional analysis of nationally representative sample. *BMJ* 324:16–19.

Shorrocks, Anthony. 1995. Revisiting the Sen poverty index. *Econometrica* 63:1225–30.

Silber, Jacques. 1982. Health and inequality: Some applications of uncertainty theory. *Social Science and Medicine* 16:1663–6.

Sitter, R.R. 1992. Comparing three bootstrap methods for survey data. *Canadian Journal of Statistics* 20:135–54.

Smedley, Brian D., Adrienne Y. Stith, and Alan R. Nelson. 2002. Unequal treatment: Confronting racial and ethnic disparities in health. Washington, DC: Institute of Medicine.

Social and economic disparities in health. 2000. Social and economic disparities in health. *Milbank Quarterly* 78 (1).

Spencer, Bruce D. 1984. Simplifying complex samples with the bootstrap. In *Proceedings of the Survey Research Methods Section*. Alexandria, VA: American Statistical Association. http//www.amstat.org/Sections/Srms/Proceedings/ (3 January 2007).

Starfield, B. 2001. Improving equity in health: A research agenda. *International Journal of Health Services* 31:545–66.

Starfield, Barbara. 2002. Equity in health. *Journal of Epidemiology and Community Health* 56:483–84.

StataCorp. 1999a. *Manual for stata statistical software: Release 6.0.* 4 vols. College Station, TX: Stata Corporation.

– 1999b. *Stata statistical software: Release 6.0.* College Station, TX: Stata Corporation.

Stoddart, Gregory L. 1995. The challenge of producing health in modern economies. *Canadian Institute for Advanced Research Population Health Working Paper* 46.

Stronks, Karien, and Louise J. Gunning-Schepers. 1993. Should equity in health be target number 1? *European Journal of Public Health* 3:104–11.

Subramanian, S.V., and Ichiro Kawachi. 2004. Income inequality and health: What have we learned so far? *Epidemiologic Review* 26:78–91.

Szwarcwald, C. Landmann. 2002. On the World Health Organisation's measurement of health inequalities. *Journal of Epidemiology and Community Health* 56:177–82.

Temkin, Larry S. 1993. *Inequality.* Oxford: Oxford University Press.

Thomas, Stephen B. 2001. The color line: Race matters in the elimination of health disparities. *American Journal of Public Health* 91:1046–8.

Thon, Dominique. 1979. On measuring poverty. *Review of Income and Wealth* 25:429–40.

– 1983. A poverty measure. *Indian Economic Journal* 30:55–70.

Tobin, James. 1970. On limiting the domain of inequality. *Journal of Law and Economics* 13:263–78.

Tsuchiya, Aki. 2000. QALYs and ageism: Philosophical theories and age weighting. *Health Economics* 9:57–68.

Tsuchiya, Aki, and Alan Williams. 2005. A 'fair innings' between the sexes: Are men being treated inequitably? *Social Science and Medicine* 60: 277–86.

Ugá, Alicia Domingues, Célia Maria de Almeida, Célia Landmann Szwarcwald, Cláudia Travassos, Francisco Viacava, José Mendes Ribeiro, Nilson do Rosário. Costa, Paulo Marchiori. Buss, and Silvia Porto. 2001. Considerations on methodology used in the World Health Organization 2000 report. *Cadernos de Saúde Pública* 17:705–12.

United Kingdom. Department of Health. 2003. Tackling health inequalities: A programme for action. http://www.dh.gov.uk/assetRoot/04/01/93/62/04019362.pdf (27 June 2006).

United Nations Development Program. 2001. Human development report 2001: Making new technologies work for human development. New York:

United Nations Development Program. http://hdr.undp.org/reports/ view_reports.cfm?type=1 (28 June 2006).

U.S. Census Bureau. 2002. *Household shares of aggregate income by fifths of the income distribution: 1967 to 2001*, 13 May 2004. http://www.census.gov/hhes/ income/histinc/ie3.html (28 June 2006).

U.S. Department of Health and Human Services. 1991. Healthy people 2000: National health promotion and disease prevention objectives. Washington, DC: U.S. Government Printing Office.

– 2000. Healthy people 2010: Understanding and improving health. Washington, DC: U.S. Government Printing Office. http://www.healthypeople.gov/ document/ (28 June 2006).

Valkonen, Tapani. 1993. Problems in the measurement and international comparisons of socio-economic differences in mortality. *Social Sciences and Medicine* 36:409–18.

Van de Vathorst, Suzanne, and Carlos Alvarez-Dardet. 2000. Doctors as judges: The verdict on responsibility for health. *Journal of Epidemiology and Community Health* 54:162–4.

Van Doorslaer, Eddy, and Xander Koolman. 2004. Explaining the differences in income-related health inequalities across European countries. *Health Economics* 13:609–28.

Veatch, R.M. 1991. Justice and the right to health care: An egalitarian account. In *Rights to Health Care*, ed. Bole, T.J. and W.B. Bonderson. Dordrecht, Netherlands: Kluwer.

Veatch, Robert. 1988. Justice and the economics of terminal illness. *Hastings Center Report* 18:34–40.

Vonnegut, Kurt, Jr. 1950. Harrison Bergeron. In *Welcome to the Monkey House*. Delacorte Press.

Wagstaff, Adam. 2001. Economics, health and development: Some ethical dilemmas facing the World Bank and the international community. *Journal of Medical Ethics* 27:262–7.

– 2002a. Inequality aversion, health inequalities and health achievement. *Journal of Health Economics* 21:627–41.

– 2002b. Poverty and health sector inequalities. *Bulletin of the World Health Organization* 80:97–105.

– 2005. Inequality decomposition and geographic targeting with applications to China and Vietnam. *Health Economics* 14:649–53.

Wagstaff, Adam, and Eddy van Doorslaer. 2000. Income inequality and health: What does the literature tell us? *Annual Review of Public Health* 21:543–67.

– 2004. Overall versus socioeconomic health inequality: A measurement framework and two empirical illustrations. *Health Economics* 13:297–301.

Wagstaff, Adam, Pierella Paci, and Eddy van Doorslaer. 1991. On the measurement of inequalities in health. *Social Science and Medicine* 33:545–57.

Walzer, Michael. 1983. *Spheres of justice.* New York: Basic Books.

Ware, John E., Jr, Robert H. Brook, Allyson R. Davies, and Kathleen N. Lohr. 1981. Choosing measures of health status for individuals in general populations. *American Journal of Public Health* 71:620–5.

Warner, Geoffrey. 2001. A Lorenz Curve based index of income stratification. *Review of Black Political Economy* Winter:41–57.

Weinick, Robin M., and Samuel H. Zuvekas. 2000. Racial and ethnic differences in access to and use of health care services, 1977 to 1996. *Medical Care Research and Review* 57:36–54.

Whitehead, Margaret. 1992. The concepts and principles of equity and health. *International Journal of Health Services* 22:429–45.

Why rank countries. 2001. Why rank countries by health performance? *The Lancet* 357:1633.

Wikler, Daniel. 1987. Personal responsibility for illness. In *Health Care Ethics: An Introduction,* ed. D. VanDeVeer and T. Regan. Philadelphia: Temple University Press.

– 1997. Bioethics, human rights, and the renewal of health for all: An Overview. In *Ethics, Equity and the Renewal of WHO's Health-for-all Strategy,* ed. Z. Bankowski, J.H. Bryant, and J. Gallagher. Geneva: CIOMS (Council for International Organizations of Medical Sciences).

– 2004. Personal and social responsibility for health. In *Public health, ethics, and equity,* ed. S. Anand, F. Peter, and A. Sen. Oxford: Oxford University Press.

Wilkins, Russell, Jean-Marie Berthelot, and Edward Ng. 2002. Trends in mortality by neighbourhood income in urban Canada from 1971 to 1996. *Supplement to Health Reports* 13:45–72. http://www.statcan.ca/bsolc/english/ bsolc? catno=82-003-S20020016353 (28 June 2006).

Wilkinson, Richard G. 1996. *Unhealthy societies: The afflictions of inequality.* London: Routledge.

Wilkinson, Richard G., and Kate E. Pickett. 2006. Income inequality and population health: A review and explanation of the evidence. *Social Science and Medicine* 62:1768–84.

Williams, Alan. 1997a. Intergenerational equity: An exploration of the 'fair innings' argument. *Health Economics* 6:117–32.

– 1997b. Conceptual and empirical issues in the efficiency-equity trade-off in the provision of health care or, if we are going to get a fair innings, someone will need to keep the score! In *Being Reasonable about the Economics of Health: Selected Essays by Alan Williams,* ed. A.J. Culyer and A. Maynard. Cheltenham, UK: Edward Elgar.

– 2001. Science or marketing at WHO? A commentary on 'World Health 2000.' *Health Economics* 10:93–100.

Williams, Alan, and Richard Cookson. 2000. Equity in health. In *Handbook of Health Economics*, ed. A.J. Culyer and J.P. Newhouse. Amsterdam: Elsevier Science.

Williams, Ruth F.G., and Darrel P. Doessel. 2006. Measuring inequality: Tools and an illustration. *International Journal for Equity in Health* 5. http://www.equity healthj.com/content/5/1/5 (28 June 2006).

Wolfson, Michael, and Geoff Rowe. 2001. On measuring inequalities in health. *Bulletin of the World Health Organization* 79:553–60.

Woodward, Alistair, and Ichiro Kawachi. 2000. Why reduce health inequalities? *Journal of Epidemiology and Community Health* 54:923–9.

– 2001. Why should physicians be concerned about health inequalities? Because inequalities are unfair and hurt everyone. *Western Journal of Medicine* 175:6–7.

World Bank. 2006. *PovertyNet*. http://web.worldbank.org/WBSITE/EXTERNAL /TOPICS/EXTPOVERTY/0,menuPK:336998~pagePK:149018~piPK: 149093~theSitePK:336992,00.html (28 June 2006).

World Health Organization. 1946. Preamble to the constitution of the World Health Organization as adopted by the international health conference, New York, 19–22 June 1946, signed on 22 July 1946 by the representatives of 61 states and entered into force on 7 April 1948. *Official Records of the World Health Organization* 2.

– 2000a. The World Health Report 2000: Health systems: Improving perform-ance. Geneva: World Health Organization. http://www.who.int/whr/en/ (28 June 2006).

– 2000b. *World Health Survey, short version questionnaire, rotation A.2.1–2.2*, 16 September 2003. http://www3.who.int/whs/P/instrumentandrel8293 .html (28 June 2006).

– 2001. *International classification of functioning, disability and health*. Geneva: World Health Organization.

– 2004. The World Health Report 2004: Changing history. Geneva: World Health Organization. http://www.who.int/whr/en/ (28 June 2006).

– 2006. *Commission on Social Determinants of Health*, http://www.who.int/social_ determinants/en/ (28 June 2006).

Xu, Kuan, and Lars Osberg. 2001. How to decompose the Sen-Shorrocks-Thon Poverty index: A practitioner's guide. *Journal of Income Distribution* 10:77–94.

Yao, Shujie. 1999. On the decomposition of Gini coefficients by population class and income source: A spreadsheet approach and application. *Applied Economics* 31:1249–64.

Yitzhaki, Shlomo. 1983. On an extension of the Gini index. *International Economic Review* 24:617–28.

– 1994. Economic distance and overlapping of distributions. *Journal of Econometrics* 61:147–59.

Yitzhaki, Shlomo, and Robert I. Lerman. 1991. Income stratification and income inequality. *Review of Income and Wealth* 37:313–29.

Young, Iris Marion. 1990. *Justice and the politics of difference*. Princeton, NJ: Princeton University Press.

– 2001. Equality of whom? Social groups and judgments of injustice. *Journal of Political Philosophy* 9:1–18.

Zheng, Buhong. 2001. Testing Lorenz Curves with non-simple random samples. *Econometrica* 70:1235–43.

Index

health inequality index, 104,
132, 210, 239n20, 255n2
on health expectation, 62, 63, 64,
89, 90, 92
on intermediate inequality, 121,
211, 213, 215
on methodological aspects of unit
of analysis, 87, 88
on moral aspects of unit of analysis, 16, 83, 197
on the moral perspective of the
WHO health inequality
index, 42, 43, 44, 63
on the probability density function, 223
on unit of analysis, 11, 16, 81,
197
on *The World Health Report 2000*,
15, 239n20
gender
definition of, 35
empirical results of, 168–70, 184,
186
example of, 43–4
in *Healthy People 2010*, 84
and the Shortfalls in Achievement, 254n6
gene. *See* genetics
generalized Concentration Index.
See Concentration Index
genetics, 34–5, 42, 240n3, 241n10,
243n6
and health expectation, 64
See also chance
geographic location, 81, 165, 191
in *Healthy People 2010*, 84, 190
Gini coefficient
and aggregation, 111, 113
applied for health in other
studies, 9–10, 185, 188,
192–4

as an attractive health inequality
measure, 132, 145–6, 198,
and comparison, 108
definition of, 107, 147, 209–10
extended, 112–13, 247n17,
248n19
as a selected health inequality
measure, 104–6, 130
statistical inference of, 148, 223–4
subgroup decomposition of,
128–9, 131, 146–50, 224–6,
256n10
Goldman, Noreen, 13
Graham, Hilary, 247n15
group approach. *See* unit of analysis
growth hormone, 59
Gunning-Schepers, Louise, 13, 15
Gwatkin, Davidson, 241n9

HALex (Health and Activity Limitation Index), construction of,
142–5
HALYs (Health-Adjusted Life Years),
discussion of, 93–4
'Harrison Bergeron,' 4
Hausman, Dan, 29, 40–1
head-count ratio, 151–2, 177, 227–8,
229–30, 256n13
health
definition of, 54
determinants of. *See* social determinants of health
as functionality, 54–9
the minimally adequate level of.
See minimally adequate level
of health
as a natural good, 11, 23
as a social good, 23
health behaviour, 31–2, 33–8. *See also*
choice, lifestyle; responsibility
Health Canada, 5